Smoothie Detox Reset Challenge

Smoothie Detox Reset Challenge

Your road to better health and permanent weight loss

By Immacula Oligario

October 25, 2022

To contact the publisher, visit WWW.YESICANSEMINARS.COM

To contact the author, visit WWW.YESICANSEMINARS.COM

ISBN: 979-8-9879884-0-4

Printed in the United States of America

Dedication

I am dedicating this book
to the memory of my late mother,
Josette Nicolas Oligario,
and to all of those who,
like me,
at some point have struggled with food.
To the sweet spirit
of my angel
Shani Duplessy,
you are gone,
but not forgotten.
To my newly departed angel
Hiawatha Cromer your giving
heart helped to save my life
which allowed me to see my
daughter get married,
create lasting
memories with my
grandchildren.
I will always remember your
laughter, I promise to
continue to grow my
knowledge to serve and
mentor others like you.

TABLE OF CONTENTS

Acknowledgements

I would like to thank my children Genevieve Ascencio-Alcinay, (Personal photographer extraordinaire see photos on page 9 and back cover) Gilbert Ascencio Jr., Yahve Alcinay and all my other children for blessing me with your presence in this life, grandchildren Christina, Maya, Myles and Tyson for being my playmates.

Special thanks to my blessing Glenn Deans, to my friends and clients Fabienne Colimon, Florence Jean Louis Dupuy, Diana St Croix, Lucia Nixon, Marie Martin, Yasmeen Chohan, Elsie Saint Louis, Marjorie Mesidor, Crystal Cotton, Tamara House, Linda King, Keria Blue and Kenya Bradley.

Many thanks to Christian Montalvo for creating the book cover and some of the pictures inside the book, you always amaze me with your creative art style, to my assistants Kisses Matugas, Jaidine Sanchez and Mary Cris Lehitimas for their help. I could not have completed this book without you. Thank you as well to my professor and editor Lisa Pulitzer and Dr. Al Titus for putting the final touches on this work.

I want to acknowledge my mentor Hiawatha Cromer for her guidance, all my supporters, my loving friends, students and clients for their support through my journey to wellness and weight loss. I wish to thank all those who have contributed to my growth and development, and all those I have been privileged and have had the honor to contribute to their lives.

Countless Blessings.

Foreword

There are many wonderful books now available discussing values of the living foods lifestyle. Immacula Oligario's book is one of them.

In an increasingly stressful society, the ability to cope with life as well as control your weight is certainly accessible if you follow the concepts she puts forth.

Her personal experience concerning this most important subject is excellently presented.

Eating a predominantly raw foods diet heals the body at warp speed ahead bringing us back into harmony and balance.

Weight loss becomes a goal that can be accomplished and maintained easily. Pounds melt away when the body is being properly nourished.

Education is the key to success. Immacula teaches people to understand the importance of proper food choices and how they contribute to stabilizing body weight.

Her chapters are concise, to the point, and easy to understand. She connects the dots between physical, emotional and spiritual realms of existence.

Transform your life through the gift of her knowledge as she has so sincerely and beautifully written the account of her journey to abundance.

Rita Romano
Living Foods Specialist
Author of Dining in the Raw

Medical Disclaimer & Cautions

Yes I Can Seminars LLC is intended to provide general educational information. Material and workbook may not be construed as medical advice or instruction. No action or inaction should be taken based solely on the contents of this information; instead, readers should consult appropriate health professionals on any matter relating to their health and well-being.

Yes I Can Seminars, LLC does not attempt to practice medicine or provide specific medical advice, and information should not be used to make a diagnosis or to replace or overrule a qualified health care provider's judgment. Nor should users rely upon the Yes I Can Seminars LLC if they might need emergency medical treatment. We strongly encourage users to consult with a qualified health care professional for answers to personal questions. Use of programs on the Yes I Can Seminars LLC philosophy does not establish a doctor-patient relationship.

You assume full responsibility for using the information in this book, and you understand and agree that Yes I Can Seminars LLC and its affiliates are not responsible or liable for any claim, loss, or damage resulting from its use by you or any user. While we try to keep the information as accurate as possible, we disclaim any warranty concerning its accuracy, timeliness, and completeness, and any other warranty, express or implied, including warranties of.

We provide access to other websites for your convenience. Yes I Can Seminars LLC is not responsible for the availability, accuracy, or content of those external sites, nor does it endorse them. Material on the Yes I Can Seminars LLC is protected by copyright law. Permission to reprint or otherwise reproduce any document in whole or in part is prohibited, unless prior written consent is obtained from the copyright owner.

By choosing to participate at the Yes I Can Seminars LLC retreat, you acknowledge and agree to the terms of this Disclaimer and our Privacy Policy. We encourage you to read them. We reserve the right to modify these terms and policies and recommend that you periodically review them.

The information and opinions expressed here are believed to be accurate, based on the best judgment available to the author, and readers who fail to consult with appropriate health authorities assume the risk of any injuries.

WELCOME!

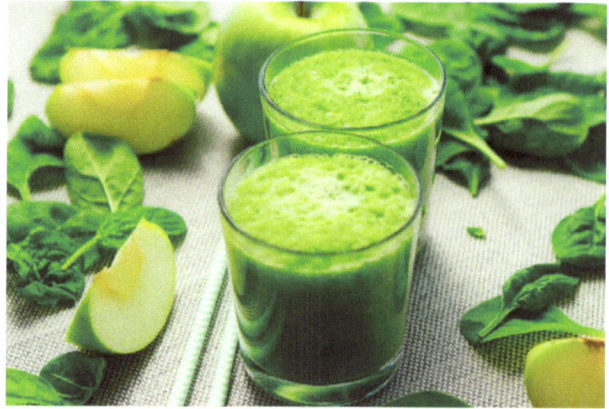

You may have heard the line, "Nothing looks as good as healthy feels." And, it's true that what can make you feel good are SIMPLE things - healthy foods and a good routine. But you might think preparing healthy meals are too complicated, and it takes so much time.

We all strive to make healthy choices in our daily lives. Unfortunately, events beyond our control occasionally disrupt our healthy habits. Maybe it was a long day at work or a stressful commute. We've all been in similar situations. Long days may result in lack of energy, emotional eating or feeling overwhelmed. It all leads to an unending downward spiral of discouragement that leads to weight gain. At times, it's hard to choose nutritious meals when you're used to eating unhealthy foods.

Today is the day that you put an end to this destructive behavior and take a step towards your vibrant health. Joining this 40-day challenge or starting a cleanse to flush toxins out of your body and break through those bothersome cravings is one of the best ways to embrace a healthy lifestyle. Green smoothies are an excellent way to jump start your weight loss, begin a wellness journey and press the "reset" button. I guarantee you that you're on the right track!

Our 40 Days Detox Smoothie Challenge includes green smoothies that are simple to make, can be customized with different flavors and toppings, and are suitable for the whole family. As you proceed through the 40 day challenge, you may begin to feel energized with a sharp mental focus. You will also feel better and be glowing! Who doesn't want to look and feel good? Well, surely not you.

I started drinking green smoothies in 2006, more than 15 years ago. I can tell you that I look and feel good even after long days of work compared to the way I felt 20 or 30 years ago. Those days, I always felt tired with low energy and a sluggish feeling. Just like you, I hired a coach who helped start me on my wellness journey in 1997.

In this book, you'll find simple, good tasting and healthy smoothie recipes created just for you. I hope you embark on this journey with an open mind. It will be worth your time, money and effort. It is my privilege and honor to have the opportunity to bring this information to you. To your health!

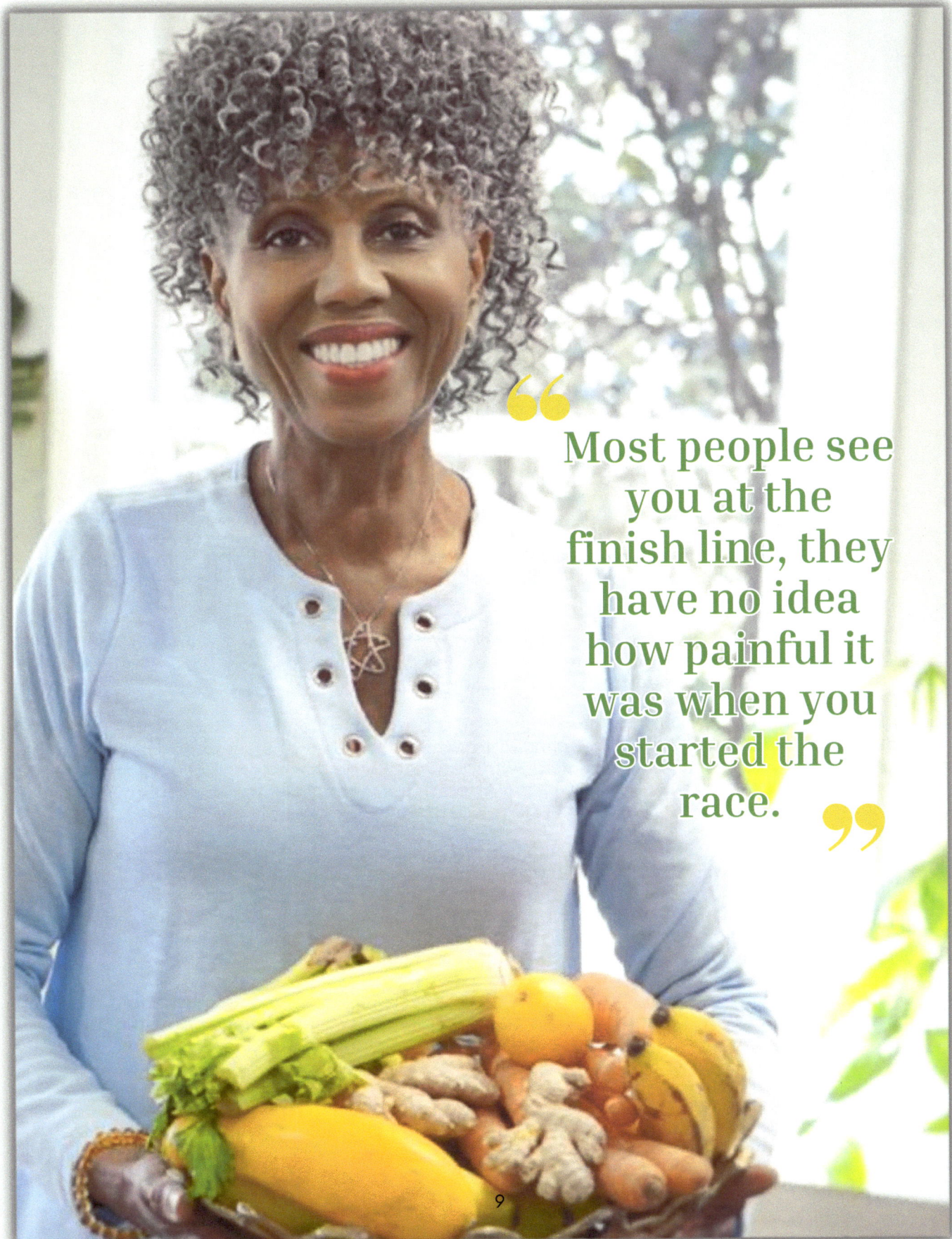

> Most people see you at the finish line, they have no idea how painful it was when you started the race.

Introduction

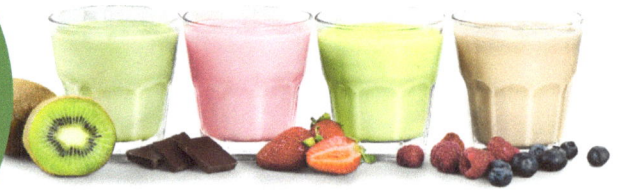

40 Day Transformational
Healthy Green Smoothie Challenge

Long before green smoothies became so popular, I was introduced to them in 2006 by my mentor, Hiawatha Cromer, a student of Dr. Ann Wigmore. In an attempt to save my life, Hiawatha told me to start blending my fruits and green leafy vegetables to help reset and improve my health. I still make smoothies a part of my daily routine.

I quickly learned that this was not just another health fad. I immediately started to feel better. Dr. Ann, as she was affectionately known, had helped many people reverse chronic, mild and debilitating diseases with smoothies. Often, her clients miraculously regained full health. She operated a health center in Boston until she made her transition in 1994.

Dr. Ann's belief was that the sun's energy had a powerful impact on green vegetation, wheatgrass and energy soup are some of the tools she used on herself and the countless clients she helped them regain optimal health.

I have an obsession with learning, influenced by my mentor Hiawatha Cromer and guided by my Blessing, Glenn. I continued to attend classes and expand my knowledge in the art and science of self-healing with nature in order to help my clients on their journey to wellness and well-being. I have offered many of my clients free healthy green smoothie recipes to "test drive" the healthy lifestyle and the benefits are many.

I decided to conduct this guided 40 Day Transformational Healthy Green Smoothie Challenge to pass on the gift I was given from the work of Dr. Ann discovery; she left behind a legacy that is still helping me, my clients, and many others. In the early '60s, Dr. Ann was helping so many people gain freedom from disease using energy soup, she was a true blessing to humanity. Later, Victoria Boutenko put the spotlight on green smoothies--which continue to open the door to self-healing.

I was inspired by the bible to do 40 days because it is said that most people who achieve success repeat the process for 30 days to embody the change of an old habit. I am not an avid reader of the bible, but I figured that to attain the Christ consciousness, 40 days of fasting preceded the enlightenment for Jesus.

I created three cycles of the 40-day challenge just with you in mind, however, you can stop when you want. I strongly recommend going through the four months to optimize your health with nutrition.

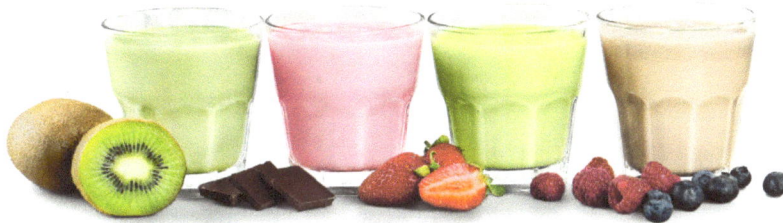

I have been on this journey for over to 16 years and the benefits are visible and tangible. My granddaughter Maya started drinking healthy green smoothies as a toddler and she sometimes ask for them. My twin grandsons just started drinking them before their first anniversary. Start them young and you don't have to worry about them turning their nose up with disdain. I cannot wait for my twin grandchildren to start asking for them by name. I did more than 152 cycles of 40 day to date. I look VIBRANT and I feel AMAZING.

I am called the **Smoothie Detox Queen** for the simple raison that my smoothies taste good and they deliver results.

I have created a cycle of three mini-series of 40 day challenges to help jumpstart your efforts.

You cannot solve obesity, prevent diseases, reset the body, or bring balance to your bodily functions using the same foods that created the problem. You first have to change the way you eat. This action will cause major shifts in the body. Also, you must start looking at your body with a truthful lens to effect real changes.

Here you have an opportunity to lose weight and keep it off for good using the method I have created. The people who have a deep desire to succeed will respond to this call and take actions that others might not.

My hope is that you would use a combination of patience and consistency, or PC, to get to your destination.

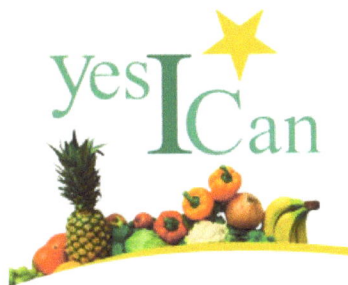

Questions and Answers

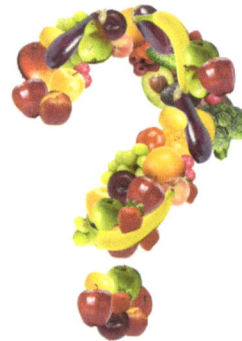

Q - Can I start anytime?
A - You can begin any time you are ready to start; we are only an email or phone call away to assist you. I would urge you to join our Facebook group because it will help stimulate you and provide valuable support when you may be hesitating or having second thoughts.

Q - How many days a week should I drink healthy green smoothies?
A - To jumpstart the body, it is important to drink 10 ounces of green smoothies four times a day and continue to eat like you did before. The introduction of the smoothies is the only change you will make in cycle one.

Q - Does a green smoothie taste good?
A - Do not let the color deter you! Smoothies have a lot of flavors, especially when herbs and sweet spices are added to them.

Q - Will the fruits increase my blood sugar?
A - Vegetables are a good way to neutralize sugar in the fruits, also adding flaxseeds or chia seeds to bulk up on fiber. Using fibrous fruits like green apples or apple pectin, cucumber and celery are good to balance out sugar in your smoothie.

Q - Will I feel full after drinking a smoothie?
A - Personally, fullness to me depends on the smoothie's thickness. Adding chia seeds and hemp heart helps me curb hunger.

Q - Are there any benefits to drinking smoothies?
A - Adapting a green smoothie lifestyle has countless benefits. After using smoothies for a long-term, many people report lower blood sugar and blood pressure, balance in their cholesterol levels, improved digestion, radiant skin, weight loss, better bowel movements, and a high energy level all day long... therefore reducing medical risks.

Q - Are green smoothies sweetened with sugar?
A - Green smoothies are to lead the foundation of a healthy lifestyle. The fact that sugar is an immune disruptor, it would be counterproductive to use sugar in the smoothie. Compared to store-bought smoothies, there's no cane sugar added to the blend. The natural sweetness of the fruits are more than enough to provide sweetness to the tasty smoothies.

Q - What age do you start to drink smoothies?
A - Smoothies are a good addition at any age from babies as soon as they are ready to transition to solid foods to geriatric care and all ages in between. However, the younger you start, the better it is.

Q - What are other benefits of drinking smoothies?
A - Drinking smoothies have many benefits. They are very alkalizing and have a powerful ability to sweep things along the intestinal tract delivering nutrients to the body, give the digestive tract a rest and detoxify the body. These are only some of the benefits.

What are Green Smoothies?

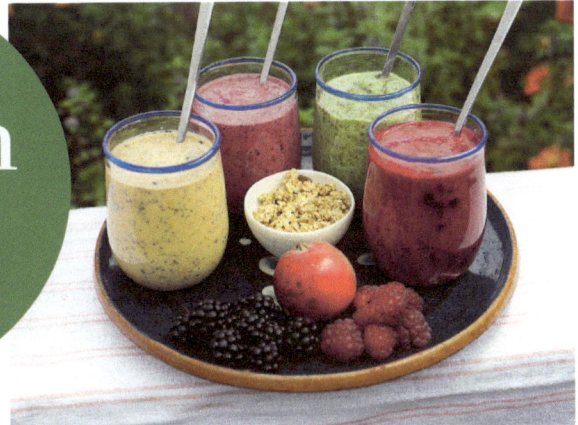

Green smoothies are known for having numerous health benefits. They are mostly green in color, being made with green vegetables and fruits. Coconut water, almond milk, coconut milk, rice milk, or plain water are liquids used to create smooth and tasty smoothies. They are loaded with vitamins from nature, and are alkalizing to the body.

Green smoothies are delicious, easy to digest, nourishing, leave you feeling satiated and full of energy. Smoothies are an easier way to consume more vegetables; dark color smoothies containing berries are usually a good way to conceal vegetables, especially for children.

Homemade green smoothies contain at least one green vegetable in addition to fruits. One word of caution: Having a commercial smoothie may provide you with more sugar than you bargained for. A 24-ounce serving of commercial smoothie may contain between 45 to 63 grams of sugar, which is not good for weight management or weight loss.

Green smoothies are great to use as meal replacements. I personally prefer them for breakfast or as late night dinner.

All you will need is a blender, water, vegetables and fruits. You can begin to transform your life in a short period of time. They are easy and fun to make, and taste amazing!

Benefits of Green Smoothies

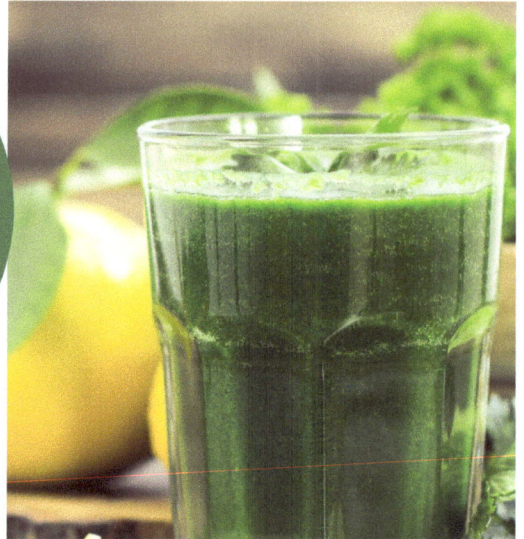

Green smoothies have numerous health benefits. Drinking green smoothies daily is a great way to add more servings of healthy fruits and vegetables into your diet. The vitamins, minerals, enzymes, phytonutrients and antioxidants contained in green smoothies can help prevent and perhaps even reverse many diseases.

Daily green smoothies are also a quick and easy way to sneak vegetables into a child's diet. Smoothies are a great way for the entire family to consume more fruits and vegetables. The American Cancer Society advise adding fruits and vegetables to your meal plan to help you stay well.

Leafy greens are a great source of vitamins and minerals and an excellent source of folate to help protect against cancer and heart disease. Smoothies are not only nutritious, they are also delicious and easy to make.

Main Benefits

The main benefits to adding green smoothie to one's diet are:

Increased fiber intake

Health promoting benefits

Natural weight loss

Inexpensive to make

Increased energy

Nutritious & Hydrating

Easy digestion & assimilation

Curb cravings

Radiant skin

Natural sugars

Mental clarity and focus

Rich in chlorophyll

Stronger hair and nails

Alkalizing to the body

Great way to hide veggies for kids

Helps eliminate toxins that make you fat

Rich in vitamins and minerals; you will require less food

Helps move food along in the intestinal tract to prevent constipation

May help stabilize blood pressure and may support balanced blood sugar

May help manage cholesterol levels

Added fiber helps you feel full, control weight without the need for dieting

To GMO or Not to GMO

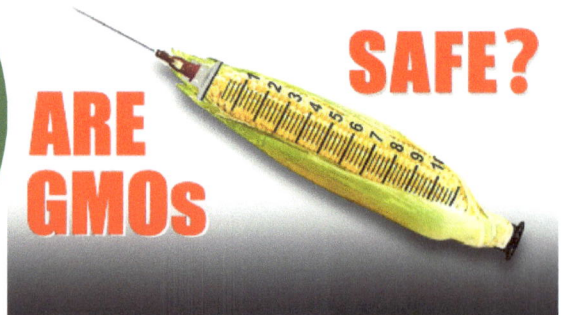

Consumer Reports, the nonprofit consumer organization, says that GMOs, or genetically modified (or engineered) organisms, are created by deliberately changing the genetic makeup of a plant, an animal, or another organism in a laboratory rather than through traditional breeding techniques. Most GMO crops currently on the market have been genetically engineered to produce their own pesticide and/or to withstand herbicides that otherwise would kill them. A generic non-GMO claim isn't reliable because there are no consistent, clear, enforceable rules for using it, and there is no consistency in how the claim is verified.

Genetically modified organisms are created in a lab by altering the genetic makeup of a plant or animal in ways that would not happen in nature. Studies in animals suggest that GMOs may cause damage to the immune system, liver, and kidneys. Animal studies commonly are used to help assess potential human health risks from exposure to substances such as synthetic chemicals and food additives.

Check out Consumer Reports at www.ConsumerReports.org for more information on GMOs, food labels, pesticides, and more. (Food safety reports and more are posted outside the paywall and available to everyone. Paid monthly or annual memberships are available if you want to read more.)

How to Read Labels

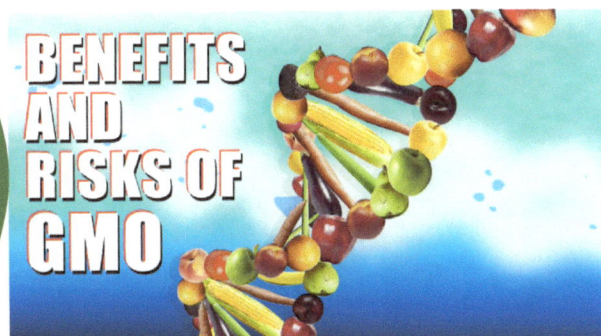

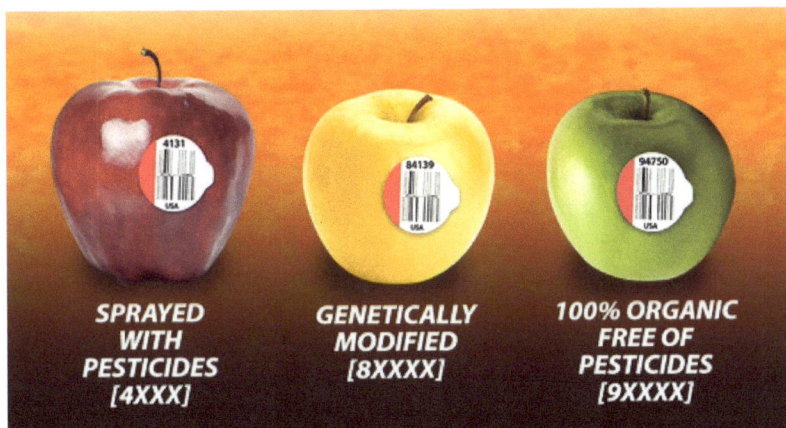

Knowing how to quickly identify conventional, organic and genetically modified produce in the store can help you ensure you go home with the best produce.

Rules for labeling fruits and vegetables in the United States aren't as stringent as they are in Europe and so it helps to know how to find the produce you're looking for.

Take a look at the numeric product codes in the image above.

The numeric code for apple on the left begins with the number 4 and has four digits on the bar code. That's the case for *all* conventional fruits and vegetables; the code begins with a 4.

The numeric code for the apple on the middle, above, begins with the number 8--meaning that it is genetically modified.

The numeric code for the apple in the right, above, begins with the number 9--meaning that it is 100 percent organic and free of pesticides.

To learn more, visit Consumer Reports at
https://www.consumerreports.org/food-labels/seals-and-claims

What EWG Has to Say

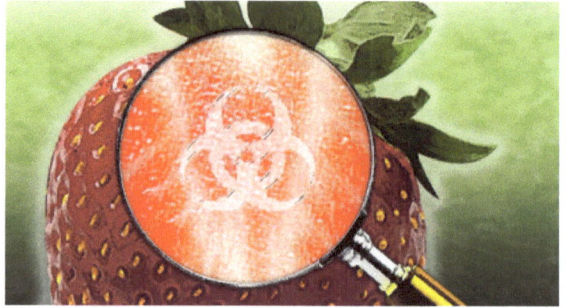

Strawberries, spinach and leafy greens are the top offenders on the Environmental Working Group's latest (2022) Dirty Dozen™ - a list of the most pesticide-contaminated fresh fruits and vegetables, based on the latest tests by the U. S. Department of Agriculture (USDA) and U. S. Food and Drug Administration (FDA).

The Dirty Dozen and the Clean Fifteen™ are EWG's lists of the most and least pesticide-contaminated conventionally grown fruits and vegetables, respectively. They are components of the annual Shopper's Guide to Pesticides in Produce™, a report EWG has released since 2004 to help consumers navigate the produce section of their grocery stores.

"Everyone should eat plenty of fresh fruit and vegetables, no matter how they're grown," said EWG Toxicologist Alexis Temkin, Ph.D. "But shoppers have the right to know what potentially toxic substances are found on these foods, so they can make the best choices for their families, given budgetary and other concerns."

Pesticide residues were found on more than 70 percent of the non-organic produce tested by the USDA and FDA. Nearly all of the levels fell *under* the legal limits allowed by government regulations. But legal does not always mean safe.

Pesticides, herbicides and certain other farm chemicals are toxic by design. Although they're meant to kill pests such as fungi, insects and plants, many pesticides are also linked to serious human health issues.

Before testing fruits and vegetables, the USDA washes, scrubs and peels them as consumers would - so it's not accurate to say that those concerned about ingesting pesticides should just wash their produce thoroughly.

"EWG recommends that, whenever possible, consumers purchase organic versions of Dirty Dozen produce," said EWG Science Analyst Sydney Swanson. "Most pesticides can't legally be applied to produce that is grown organically."

When organic options are unavailable or unaffordable, EWG advises shoppers to buy produce from its Clean Fifteen. This year, almost 70 percent of Clean Fifteen samples had no detectable pesticide residues whatsoever.

EWG's Dirty Dozen

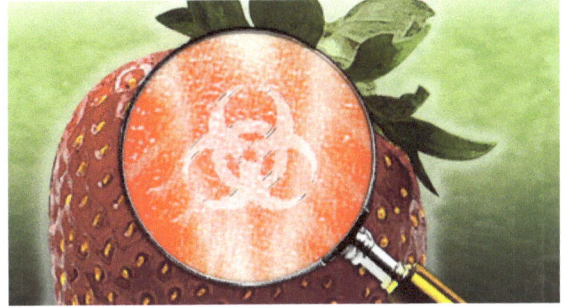

1. Strawberries
2. Spinach
3. Kale, collard & mustard greens
4. Nectarines
5. Apples
6. Grapes
7. Bell & hot peppers
8. Cherries
9. Peaches
10. Pears
11. Celery
12. Tomatoes

EWG's Clean 15

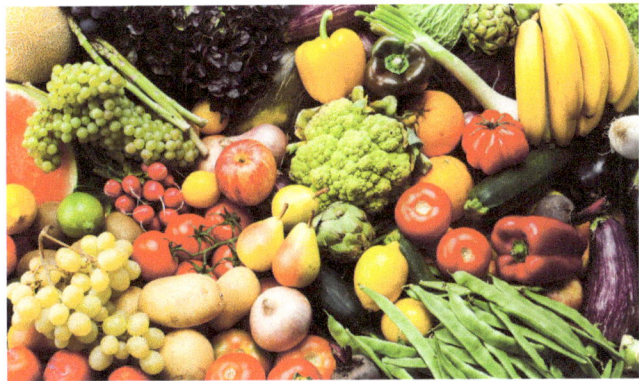

1. Avocados
2. Sweet corn
3. Pineapple
4. Onions
5. Papaya
6. Sweet peas (frozen)
7. Asparagus
8. Honeydew melon
9. Kiwi
10. Cabbage
11. Mushrooms
12. Cantaloupe
13. Mangoes
14. Watermelon
15. Sweet potatoes

Chemicals & Farm Produce

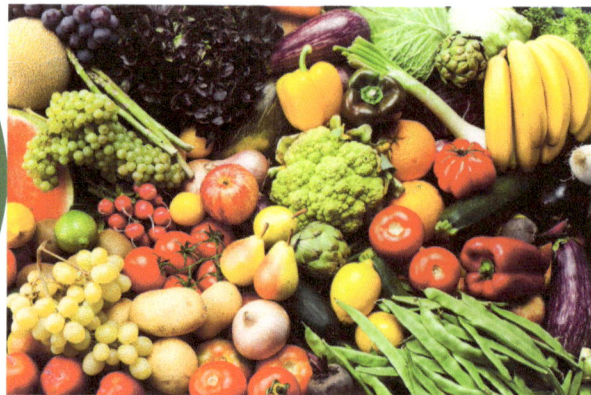

If you want to "eat clean," you will probably want to start with fruits and vegetables that are clean and free of chemicals that are often used on farm produce. These include pesticides used to destroy or prevent pests, herbicides to get rid of weeds and other unwanted vegetation, and fungicides used to halt the growth of fungi.

Farmers often rely on chemicals as they try to maximize crop yield--and there are lots of products for them to choose from.

Fortunately, groups including the non-profit Environmental Working Group and Consumer Reports have done extensive testing to help identify which ones have high chemical residues and which ones don't. Try to use the lists from these groups as you do your shopping. It's always best to go organic, but it can be expensive, so try to focus on buying organic produce when it's an important part of your diet. Consider conventional produce if it's not something that you're eating regularly.

Washing fruits and vegetables before eating them can also help reduce your exposure to chemicals. However, no wash can actually remove chemicals hidden inside the produce. That's why there's value in buying organic.

The USDA, along with the U.S. Environmental Protection Agency and Food and Drug Administration work together to monitor and set limits as to how much pesticide can be used on farms and how much is safe to remain on the product once it hits grocery store shelves.

Remember fruits and vegetables have countless health benefits; they are high in fiber, mineral and are enzymes rich. To remove pesticides from fruits and vegetables there are commercial washes available at most supermarkets or simply add 5 to 10 drops of grapefruit seed extract in one gallon of water to wash them before consumption.

Vegetables 101

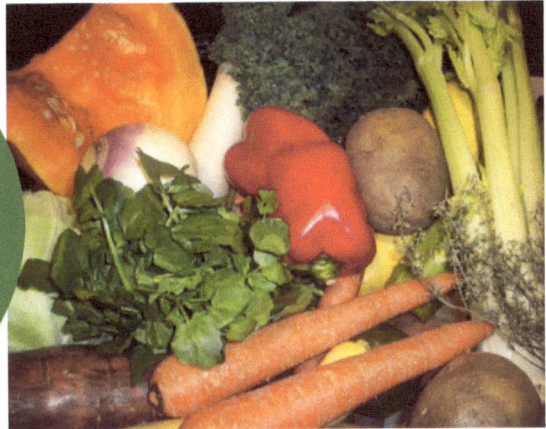

Vegetables are loaded with antioxidants, minerals and essential vitamins. No matter what the color, green, red, yellow or white, they all provide many health benefits.

Vegetables are low in fat, low in caloric intake and high in nutrients. The high fiber content in vegetables helps improve digestion. Veggies can be juiced, eaten in their raw form, canned, or kept in the freezer for later use.

It is recommended to eat at least 3 to 5 servings of vegetables a day.

It is very common to eat either steamed, stir-fried, baked, juiced, dehydrated or added to smoothies.

Vegetables are divided into into two categories: vegetables grown above ground and those grown below ground, or "root" vegetables. Here are some examples of both types:

Above ground vegetables:
- Asparagus
- Broccoli
- Cabbage
- Cauliflower
- Cucumber
- Kale
- Lettuce
- Squash
- Zucchini

Root vegetables:
- Beet
- Carrot
- Parsnip
- Radish
- Turnip

Root vegetables are a great source of carbohydrates. Vegetables grown above ground are an excellent source of phytonutrients.

Washing Fruits and Vegetables

It is important to thoroughly wash fruits and vegetables to help avoid food borne illnesses this is also a good part of prevention of diseases.

"Cleanliness is close to godliness"
-English Proverbs

You will need a colander, vegetable saver container or an ordinary rectangular plastic box, brush, knife, and stainless steel bowl big enough to hold all your fruits and vegetables.

1. Fill up a stainless steel bowl with water, add 5 drops of grapeseed fruit extract for each gallon of water.
2. Soak fruits and vegetables for 10 to 20 minutes
3. Use a brush to scrub fruits and vegetables
4. Place them in a colander to help remove excess water
5. Remove any bad spots
6. Dry fruits and vegetables
7. Place them in a plastic container
8. Refrigerate when applicable at a temperature about 34 degrees Fahrenheit

Wash solutions:

Formula 1
1. Use five drops of grapefruit seed extract for each gallon of water
2. First, soak the items intended to be washed. (Make sure storage container is free of BPA)
3. Follow with a produce brush then, rinse them either place in a strainer or use paper towel to dry before storing.

Formula 2
1. Use three tablespoons of apple cider vinegar, 1 tablespoon hydrogen peroxide, half lemon or lime can also be used
2. Soak the items intended to be washed. (Make sure storage container is free of BPA)
3. Follow with a produce brush, then rinse them. Drain them in a strainer or use a paper towel to dry before storing.

There are some fruit and vegetable washes available commercially in your health food store or regular supermarket, too.

There are many ways to wash fruits and vegetables. You have probably already guessed why it's smart to wash them: Lots of other people have already handled them. My mother said it best, "I don't know where your hands have been"

Do you know your greens?

Test Your Knowledge by Matching Names and Images

SPINACH ●   ●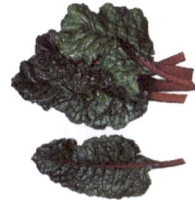

KALE ●   ●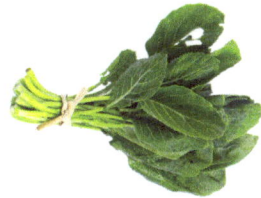

SWISS CHARD ●   ●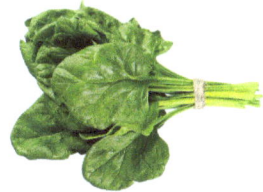

COLARD GREENS ●   ●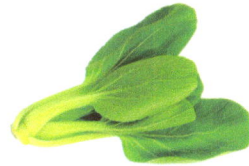

PARSLEY ●   ●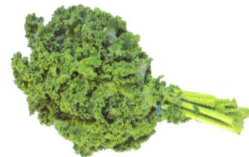

BOK CHOY ●   ●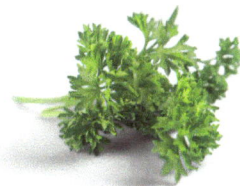

Do you know your fruits?

Test Your Knowledge by Matching Names and Images

PINEAPPLE •   •

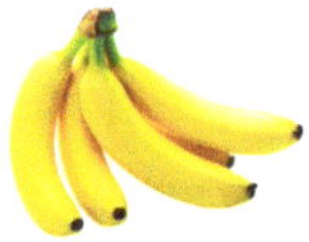

MANGO •   •

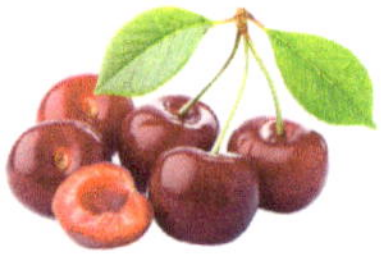

BANANA •   •

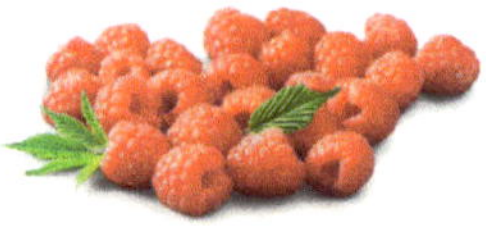

PAPAYA •   •

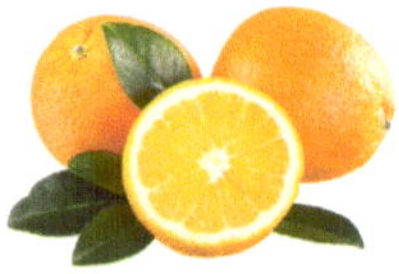

BLUEBERRY •   •

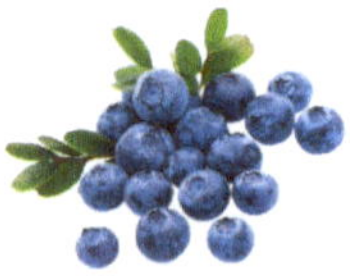

RASPBERRY •   •

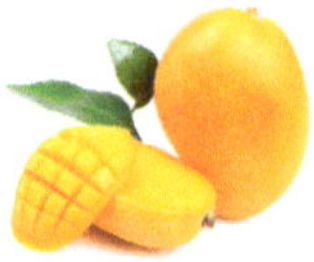

ORANGE •   •

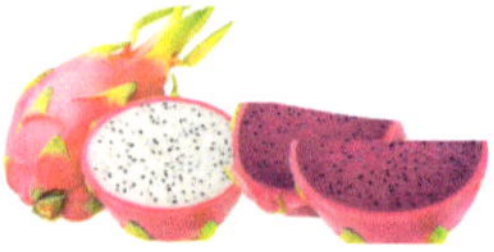

CHERRIES •   •

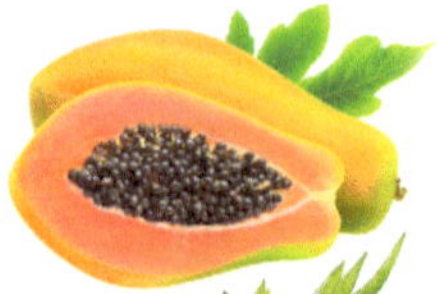

DRAGON FRUIT •   •

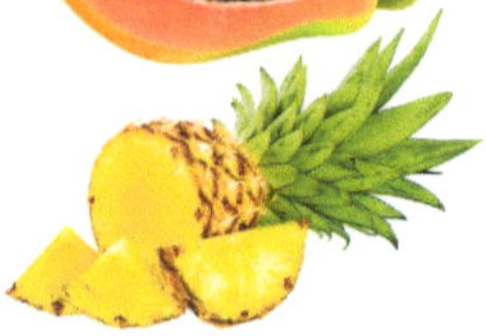

Health Benefits from Fruits and Vegetables

Spinach
- Improves Hydration
- Appetite Control
- Prevents osteoporosis
- Reduces the risk of iron deficiency anemia
- Boosts the immune system

Kale
- Great source of vitamin C
- Lowering cholesterol may reduce the risk of heart disease
- Terrific source of vitamin K
- Source of Cancer-Fighting Substances
- High Beta-Carotene Content

Swiss Chard
- Loaded with fiber
- Outstanding source of vitamin K
- May reduce blood sugar and insulin resistance
- May help with weight loss
- Heart Healthy

Collard Greens
- May help prevent cancer
- Enhances bone health
- Improves eye health
- Improves intestinal health

Parsley
- Antibacterial activities are present in parsley extract
- Easy to include in your diet
- Contains a variety of essential nutrients
- A source of antioxidants
- Helps maintain bone health

Bok Choy
- Might help thyroid function
- Maintains healthy skin
- Ensures eye health
- Help to reduce inflammation
- Reduces the risk of cardiovascular disease

Pineapple
- Contains antioxidants that fight illness
- Lowers the risk of developing cancer
- Immune system booster and anti-inflammatory agent
- May reduce arthritis symptoms
- It could help with digestion

Banana
- May benefit gastrointestinal health
- High in antioxidants
- Energy booster
- Natural laxative
- Get rid of morning sickness

Mango
- Could aid in preventing diabetes
- High concentration of beneficial plant components
- Contains nutrients that support the immune system
- May help reduce the risk of certain diseases
- Adaptable and simple to include in your diet

Papaya
- Has the potential to prevent prostate cancer
- May help reduce inflammation and help digestion
- Helps protect against heart disease
- Relieves menstrual pain

Blueberries
- Full of vitamins and minerals
- May aid in lowering cholesterol
- May aid in controlling blood sugar
- Rich in antioxidants

Raspberries
- High in nutrients
- High in antioxidants that prevent aging
- May help protect against cancer
- High in fiber

Oranges
- Citrus-rich diets may protect against chronic diseases
- Helps prevent anemia
- Might contribute to immune system health
- Help keep your eyes healthy and sharp
- Help control appetite

Cherries
- May contribute to preventing cancer
- May boost recovery from exercise
- Could help you sleep better
- May reduce the incidence of type 2 diabetes

Dragon Fruit
- Contains lots of antioxidants
- Naturally low in fat and high in fiber
- Contains prebiotics
- Can help to boost your immune system
- May increase your iron levels

Mixology

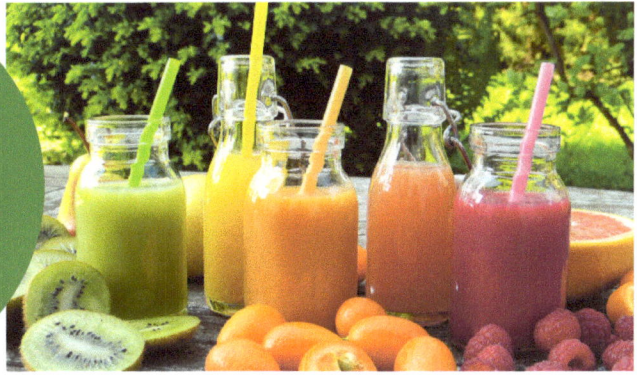

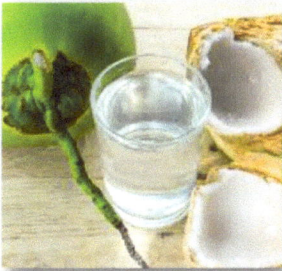

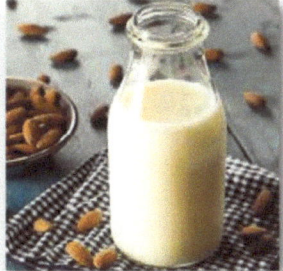

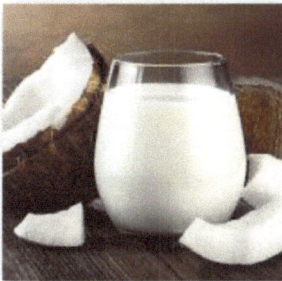

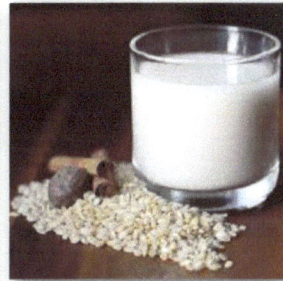

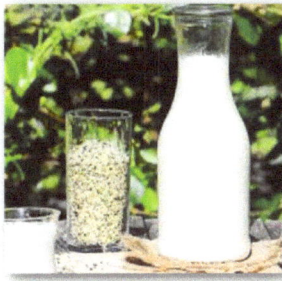

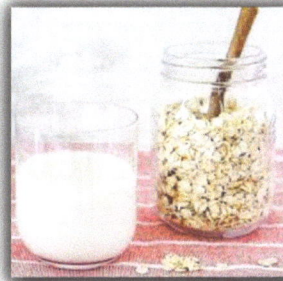

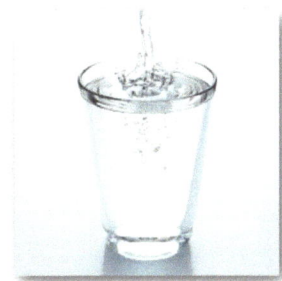

To create smooth, creamy and tasty smoothies use: coconut water, almond milk, coconut milk, rice milk, hemp milk, oat milk or plain water can be added as liquid for your mix.

Smoothie My Personal Story

Breakfast is a very important meal. You are breaking the fast from not eating while asleep when the body is working to rid itself of toxins. Most people break their overnight fast by eating heavy foods like eggs, cereals, bagel, ham, sausage, bread and cheese. However these can be very overwhelming to the body and cause symptoms like heartburn, indigestion, constipation, sluggishness, and fatigue. Try starting your day with a smoothie a day for breakfast for a week. You will quickly feel the benefits. Your energy will be doubled or tripled! That's no joke.

One green smoothie a day has all the nutrients you need to feed your body when you're on the go. Guaranteed this will make a difference. Since 2006, I have been breaking my fast with a green smoothie every morning, even when I travel. I use a portable blender when I'm on the road. No excuses.

In the beginning of my smoothie journey, I was blending daily. I was consuming more green smoothie because it was extremely challenging for my intestinal tract to process any cooked or processed foods. This was the only way for my body to receive nutrition. As years went by, I needed less food because my cells were saturated with dense nutrients from the smoothies. The blending process homogenizes the food. That allows the intestinal tract to easily extract nutrients, utilize them to feed and repair our cells, and provide energy and vitality. At first, I didn't understand where my new stamina and strength were coming from. Now, I know it was because my cells were receiving complete nutrients from the smoothies.

Over time, I have found shortcuts to help make this important lifestyle change easier and more sustainable. I want to share some of the lessons I learned along the way to help you get to the finish line. Adopting this lifestyle is a long term process and not a quick fix. Once you understand the process that fat cells go through, you can turn them off--and keep them switched off for good. Food fuels our cells and turns off cravings.

I have successfully helped countless individuals kick start their weight loss journey by simply adding 40 ounces of green smoothie to their daily food intake without making any other lifestyle changes. That one step will help you start dropping the pounds and feeling better. I have also designed three-month and six-month programs for people who need help with difficulty in weight loss. This is the same weight loss program that I used to help me slim down, maintain my weight loss, and feel better. You can achieve the same results. But you have to play fair. There can't be any excuses for you either!

Smoothie Making Tips

- Are you ready for week two? Get creative with your smoothies. Use this plan as a great foundation to build on and create something that is truly you!

- If you prefer your smoothies with a little bit of sweetness, try adding some tasty dates or dried raisins! *Remember sweet equal calories.

- Use at least one frozen fruit to make the smoothie. Or, you can add ice cubes to the blender to keep it chilled.

Prepare several days worth of smoothies and keep them in the refrigerator. This will help you stay consistent with your plan.

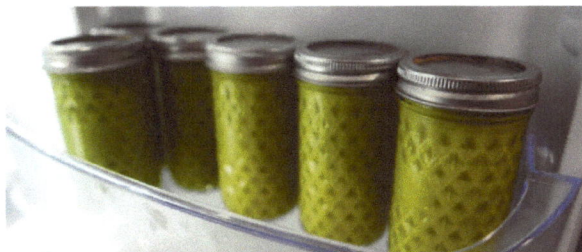

- Preparing all your smoothies ahead of time will make it easier for you to stick with your plan, especially when you're short on time!

- Are you putting in long days at work? No problem. Make your smoothie the night before and have it ready and waiting for you in the fridge when it's time to go.

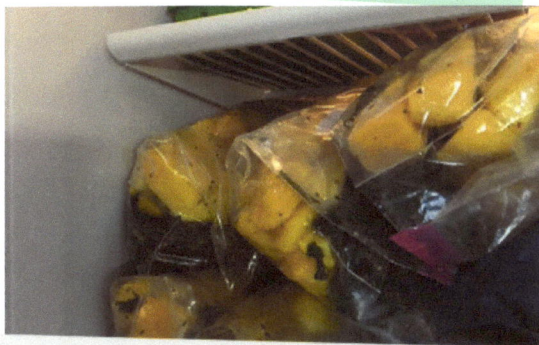

Save time by prepping your smoothie ingredients in advance. Bag them, and toss the bags in the freezer.

Consider storing your smoothies in a glass mason jar to help avoid chemicals found in some plastics. See next page for more information on BPA

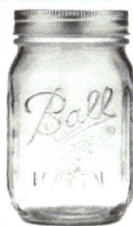

When you're ready to make your smoothies, grab a bag from the freezer. Add water and blend. Voila! You're done.

BPA Safety

Remember to keep things clean and free of toxins at every step of the way-and that includes how you store that delicious green smoothie that you just created from fresh ingredients. Plastic food containers can contain a chemical called BPA, or bisphenol A.

You can avoid the chemical either by buying and storing your smoothies in BPA-free containers or (better yet) glass containers.

Some studies have linked BPA to an elevated risk of health issues, such as fertility problems and certain cancers, but it remains widely used to harden plastic, prevent metal corrosion, and coat paper. It can be found in hard-plastic water bottles, though more companies are offering BPA-free alternatives because of the health concerns.

The Endocrine Society, which represent thousands of physicians and scientists who specialize in hormone-related disorders, says that studies have linked low levels of BPA and similar chemicals to problems with reproduction, metabolism, and behavior. The American Academy of Pediatrics has cautioned that BPA "can act like estrogen in the body and potentially change the timing of puberty, decrease fertility, increase body fat, and affect the nervous and immune systems."

BPA is what's known as an endocrine disruptor, which means that it can interfere with or mimic the actions of your hormones. Such disruptions can have effects throughout the body.

To learn more, visit Consumer Reports at https://www.consumerreports.org/bpa/bpa-exposure-may-be-much-greater-than-previously-believed/

More information on plastic safety from noted Professor Paul Knoepfler, Ph.D, can be found at https://ipscell.com/2012/03/helpful-concise-guide-to-safe-use-of-plastics/

Picking Your Blender

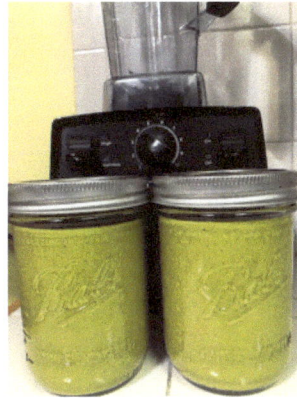

Any blender is a great start as long as you can make your smoothie to support your ultimate well-being!

Committing to having a daily green smoothie as a lifestyle is not an easy decision to make, if what you have known all your life is the Standard American Diet. This change doesn't have to come with a high ticket price, making it more difficult to achieve.

To get started, try using the equipment and utensils that you have at home. See how things go and gauge your level of interest. Is this something you want to do over the long term or not? Once you've decided what path you want to take, then consider what you really need to optimize your time in the kitchen. I tested my personal commitment to improve my health for six months before purchasing an expensive high speed blender.

I used an Oster brand blender to make my smoothies in the beginning, because that was the brand I owned. It worked well enough to get me going. I felt the difference drinking my smoothie quiet quickly. My energy level went up, and my digestive system was happier, too. Eventually, I decided to step up to a better (and more expensive) VitaMix blender. This new blender made a difference; my smoothies were creamy, smooth, and more enjoyable. The blender made a world of difference in both texture and speed.

For close to two decades I have been blending my breakfast with the same blender. VitaMix has a warranty policy that is exceptional. When my blender stopped working after 13 years, it was repaired at no cost to me. I was already sold on the equipment, but now, I was   enchanted with their customer service.

Know that this small step of blending fruits and vegetables can add years to your life.

For more information on blenders, please see the Resource Section below on page 79

Daily Planner

1-14-2022

TOP PRIORITIES

Weightloss

Get physical to prevent diseases

Spend quality time with family

Be productive at work/ financial freedom

TODAY'S SCHEDULE

6-7 AM	Drink water
7-8 AM	Drink water
8-9 AM	Drink water
9-10 AM	Go to work
10-11 AM	Drink water
11-12 AM	Smoothie
12-1 PM	Lunch
1-2 PM	Drink water
2-3 PM	Smoothie
3-4 PM	Drink water
4-5 PM	Smoothie
6-7 PM	Dinner
7-8 PM	Smoothie
8-9 PM	Self-care

TO DO LIST..

- [ ] Shop for green smoothie ingredients
- [ ] Learn about personal development
- [ ] Create a vision board
- [ ] Invest in a good blender
- [ ] Drink water

FOR TOMORROW..

Get physical to prevent diseases

SELF-CARE

5-minute meditation.
Take a lavender bath
Watch a comedy movie

GRATITUDE

Grateful for my health
My bodily functions
For fulfilling career
Helping hands

ACTION AND OUTCOME

Add four green smoothies a day → Lighter and more energy
Invite my sister over for dinner. → Strengthen our bond
Learn to delegate at work. → To show my leadership skills

NOTE..

Today was a very good day,
I learned a lot about myself.
I feel more energized.

WATER - ✓✓✓✓✓✓✓✓✓✓✓✓

SMOOTHIE - ✓✓✓✓✓✓✓✓

Download a blank copy of the Daily Planner from
www.yesicanseminars.com

Self-care: What Experts Say

"It's not selfish to love yourself, take care of yourself, and to make your happiness a priority. It's necessary".

- Mandy Hale

" When you say "yes" to others make sure you are not saying "no" to yourself."

- Paulo Coehlo

"Self-care is not self-indulgence, it is self-preservation."

- Audre Lorde

"Self-care is how you take your power back. "

- Lalah Delia

"Self-care is giving the world the best of you instead of what's left of you."

-Katie Reed

"Rest and self-care are so important. When you take time to replenish your spirit, it allows you to serve from the overflow. You cannot serve from an empty vessel."

-Eleanor Brown

40-day Self-care

① ✔ Place a check mark in the box

① Learn to meditate ☐	② Drink water ☐	③ Go to bed early ☐	④ Walk in nature ☐	⑤ Put yourself first ☐	⑥ Find moments of gratitude ☐
⑦ Organize your space ☐	⑧ Listen to music ☐	⑨ Watch a comedy movie ☐	⑩ Set your short term and long term goals ☐	⑪ Take a break from social media ☐	⑫ Sign up for a free yoga class ☐
⑬ Spend quality time with family ☐	⑭ Rest ☐	⑮ Go to bed an hour earlier ☐	⑯ Laugh out loud ☐	⑰ Watch the sunrise ☐	⑱ Take a long bath ☐
⑲ Eat healthy meals ☐	⑳ Sing more often ☐	㉑ Get some fresh air ☐	㉒ Write your journal ☐	㉓ Take a deep breath ☐	㉔ Drink smoothies ☐
㉕ Take a lavender bath ☐	㉖ Get extra sleep ☐	㉗ Create a vision board ☐	㉘ Take a break from a toxic situation ☐	㉙ Create a bucket list ☐	㉚ Take a nap ☐
㉛ Be adventurous ☐	㉜ Forgive yourself and others ☐	㉝ Have a quiet time ☐	㉞ Get a facial ☐	㉟ Get a body massage ☐	㊱ Be compassionate to yourself ☐
㊲ Let go of the past ☐	㊳ Commit to a self-improvement ☐	㊴ Watch the sunset ☐	㊵ Exercise ☐	👏 ☐	🥤 ☐

Download a blank copy of the Self-Care chart from
www.yesicanseminars.com

40-day Self Care

Self care is not being selfish as we may believe it to be. It's our ability to ask for help, to say no, or to set boundaries. It can be compared to when traveling by plane and the flight attendant ask you to put you mask on first before helping someone else even when traveling with an infant, it is self preservation.

It is okay to put yourself first by doing that you will have more to give, self care is doing something for you, like exercising, choosing healthy meals or extra sleep to promote good health.

If you run out of self care ideas we have provided a list from the previous page as a guideline for your self care needs, please feel free to write daily in the box numbered for your convenience.

Variety creates excitement. We encourage you to explore something new daily, diversity is good to help foster change, sameness may encourage boredom this may result in self sabotage.

Daily Journal

Consistency is the key to success!

SAMPLE

1	DATE: Feb28
	DAY: Tue

MANGO SUNSHINE ✓

1	DATE: _____ DAY: _____

MANGO SUNSHINE ☐

2	DATE: _____ DAY: _____

MANGO SUNSHINE ☐

3	DATE: _____ DAY: _____

ISLAND KALE ☐

4	DATE: _____ DAY: _____

ISLAND KALE ☐

5	DATE: _____ DAY: _____

GLORIOUS GREEN ☐

6	DATE: _____ DAY: _____

GLORIOUS GREEN ☐

7	DATE: _____ DAY: _____

SUN KISSED STRAWBERRY ☐

8	DATE: _____ DAY: _____

SUN KISSED STRAWBERRY ☐

9	DATE: _____ DAY: _____

SMOOTH SUNSET ☐

10	DATE: _____ DAY: _____

SMOOTH SUNSET ☐

11	DATE: _____ DAY: _____

PINEAPPLE SURPRISE ☐

12	DATE: _____ DAY: _____

PINEAPPLE SURPRISE ☐

13	DATE: _____ DAY: _____

VERY CHERRY BERRY GARDEN ☐

14	DATE: _____ DAY: _____

VERY CHERRY BERRY GARDEN ☐

15	DATE: _____ DAY: _____

GONE BANANAS ☐

16	DATE: _____ DAY: _____

GONE BANANAS ☐

17	DATE: _____ DAY: _____

FLOWING MOVEMENT ☐

18	DATE: _____ DAY: _____

FLOWING MOVEMENT ☐

19	DATE: _____ DAY: _____

PINEAPPLE ORANGE ON THE GREEN ☐

20	DATE: _____ DAY: _____

PINEAPPLE ORANGE ON THE GREEN ☐

21	DATE: _____ DAY: _____

PINA COLADA ON THE GREEN ☐

22	DATE: _____ DAY: _____

PINA COLADA ON THE GREEN ☐

23	DATE: _____ DAY: _____

VERY BERRY MOUSSE ☐

24	DATE: _____ DAY: _____

VERY BERRY MOUSSE ☐

25	DATE: _____ DAY: _____

TROPICAL EXPLOSION ☐

26	DATE: _____ DAY: _____

PURPLE BLINDDATE ☐

27	DATE: _____ DAY: _____

BLUEBERRY PASSION ☐

28	DATE: _____ DAY: _____

TROPICAL SENSES ☐

29	DATE: _____ DAY: _____

TROPICAL GREENS ☐

30	DATE: _____ DAY: _____

COCONUT BREEZE ☐

31	DATE: _____ DAY: _____

GREEN APPLE PIE ☐

32	DATE: _____ DAY: _____

MANGO MELLOW ☐

33	DATE: _____ DAY: _____

MANGO FRESCA ☐

34	DATE: _____ DAY: _____

MANGO TONIC ☐

35	DATE: _____ DAY: _____

MANGO TONIC FRESCA ☐

36	DATE: _____ DAY: _____

PAPAYA TONIC ☐

37	DATE: _____ DAY: _____

GONE BANANA TONIC ☐

38	DATE: _____ DAY: _____

PINEAPPLE TONIC ☐

39	DATE: _____ DAY: _____

PINEAPPLE FRESCA ☐

40	DATE: _____ DAY: _____

CARIBBEAN ALL SPICE ☐

Download a blank copy of the Daily Planner chart from www.yesicanseminars.com

Track Your Favorites

40 DAYS *Smoothie Detox Reset Challenge*

Tracking Your Favorites

Create a lifestyle with your favorites!

Encircle:

🥰 Love it!

😊 It's okay

☹️ I don't like it

1 MANGO SUNSHINE 🥰 😊 ☹️	**2** MANGO SUNSHINE 🥰 😊 ☹️	**3** ISLAND KALE 🥰 😊 ☹️
4 ISLAND KALE 🥰 😊 ☹️	**5** GLORIOUS GREEN 🥰 😊 ☹️	**6** GLORIOUS GREEN 🥰 😊 ☹️
7 SUN KISSED STRAWBERRY 🥰 😊 ☹️	**8** SUN KISSED STRAWBERRY 🥰 😊 ☹️	**9** SMOOTH SUNSET 🥰 😊 ☹️
10 SMOOTH SUNSET 🥰 😊 ☹️	**11** PINEAPPLE SURPRISE 🥰 😊 ☹️	**12** PINEAPPLE SURPRISE 🥰 😊 ☹️
13 VERY CHERRY BERRY GARDEN 🥰 😊 ☹️	**14** VERY CHERRY BERRY GARDEN 🥰 😊 ☹️	**15** GONE BANANAS 🥰 😊 ☹️
16 GONE BANANAS 🥰 😊 ☹️	**17** FLOWING MOVEMENT 🥰 😊 ☹️	**18** FLOWING MOVEMENT 🥰 😊 ☹️
19 PINEAPPLE ORANGE ON THE GREEN 🥰 😊 ☹️	**20** PINEAPPLE ORANGE ON THE GREEN 🥰 😊 ☹️	**21** PINA COLADA ON THE GREEN 🥰 😊 ☹️
22 PINA COLADA ON THE GREEN 🥰 😊 ☹️	**23** VERY BERRY MOUSSE 🥰 😊 ☹️	**24** VERY BERRY MOUSSE 🥰 😊 ☹️
25 TROPICAL EXPLOSION 🥰 😊 ☹️	**26** PURPLE BLIND DATE 🥰 😊 ☹️	**27** BLUEBERRY PASSION 🥰 😊 ☹️
28 TROPICAL SENSES 🥰 😊 ☹️	**29** TROPICAL GREENS 🥰 😊 ☹️	**30** COCONUT BREEZE 🥰 😊 ☹️
31 GREEN APPLE PIE 🥰 😊 ☹️	**32** MANGO MELLOW 🥰 😊 ☹️	**33** MANGO FRESCA 🥰 😊 ☹️
34 MANGO TONIC 🥰 😊 ☹️	**35** MANGO TONIC FRESCA 🥰 😊 ☹️	**36** PAPAYA TONIC 🥰 😊 ☹️
37 GONE BANANA TONIC 🥰 😊 ☹️	**38** PINEAPPLE TONIC 🥰 😊 ☹️	**39** PINEAPPLE FRESCA 🥰 😊 ☹️
40 CARIBBEAN ALL SPICE 🥰 😊 ☹️	👏	🥤🥦

Download a blank copy of the Daily Planner chart from
www.yesicanseminars.com

Healthy Lifestyle Tips

AVOID microwave vegetables since this process zaps the nutrients and they become void of nourishment. The food is dead; it has no nutritional value and leaves the body starving for nutrition.

AVOID canned goods, they are loaded with a significant amount of salt and sugar to help preserve the canned goods.
EAT a variety of fruits and vegetables to get a full range of vitamins and minerals

MANGO SUNSHINE

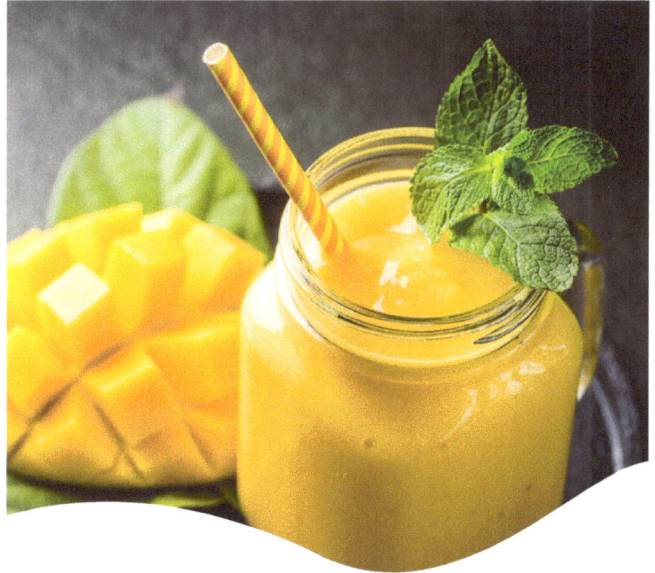

INGREDIENTS

1 cup spinach
1 cup coconut milk
1 orange
1 ½ cup mango

DIRECTIONS

Place everything into the blender along with water and blend until smooth.

ISLAND KALE

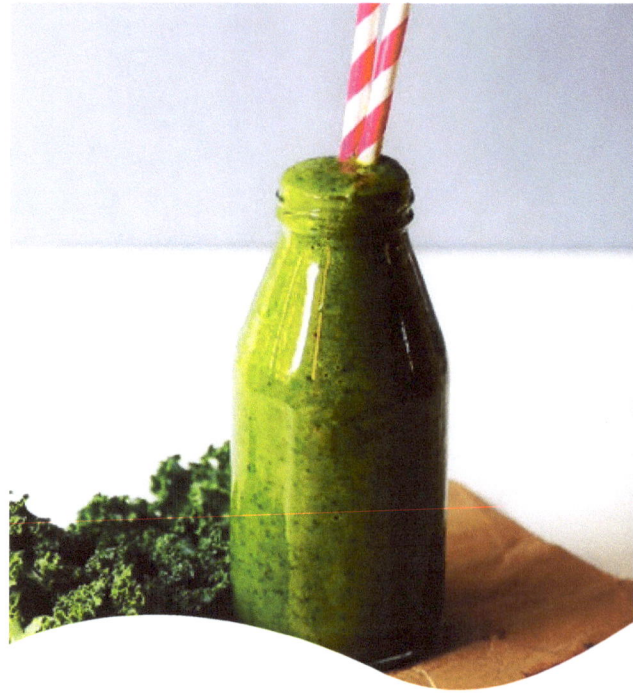

INGREDIENTS

1 cup kale

1 cup water

1/2 cup pineapples

1/2 cup strawberries

1 banana

1/4 teaspoon cinnamon

DIRECTIONS

Place everything into the blender along with water and blend until smooth.

GLORIOUS GREEN

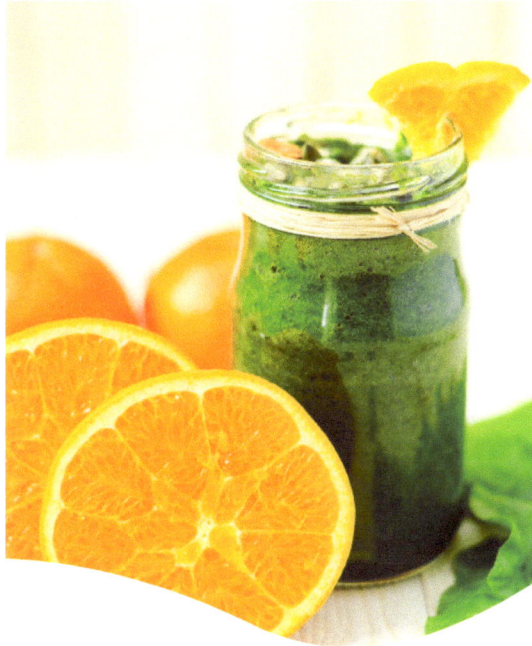

INGREDIENTS

1 cup spinach
1 cup water
1 orange
1 cup pineapple
1/2 banana

DIRECTIONS

Place everything into the blender along with water and blend until smooth.

SUN KISSED STRAWBERRY

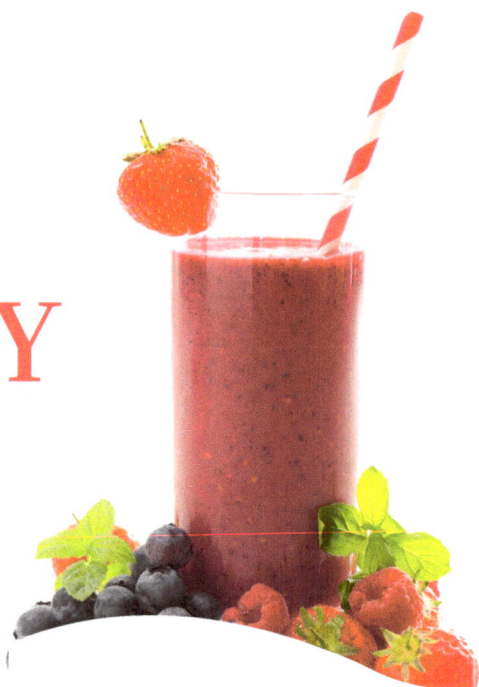

INGREDIENTS

1 cup spinach

1 cup water

1 orange

1 ½ cup strawberries

DIRECTIONS

Place everything into the blender along with water and blend until smooth.

SMOOTH SUNSET

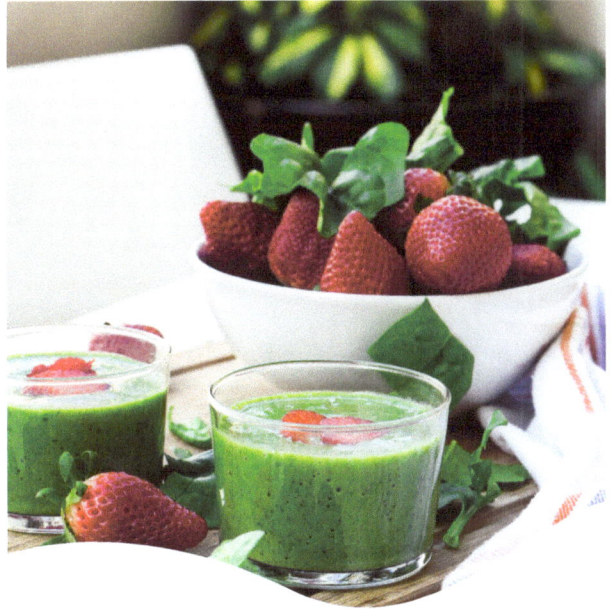

INGREDIENTS

1 cup spinach

3 leaves of basil

1 cup water

1 cup mango

1 ½ cup strawberries

DIRECTIONS

Place all ingredients in a blender,
process until smooth

PINEAPPLE SURPRISE

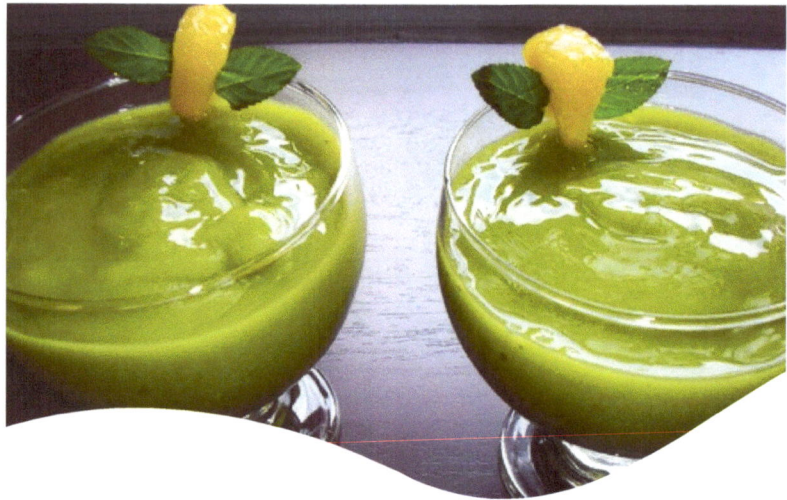

INGREDIENTS

1 whole pineapple
1 bunch of spinach
1 ½ cup of water

DIRECTIONS

Wash spinach thoroughly
Peel pineapple and cut into chunks
Place all ingredients in a blender
Cover and process until smooth

VERY CHERRY BERRY GARDEN

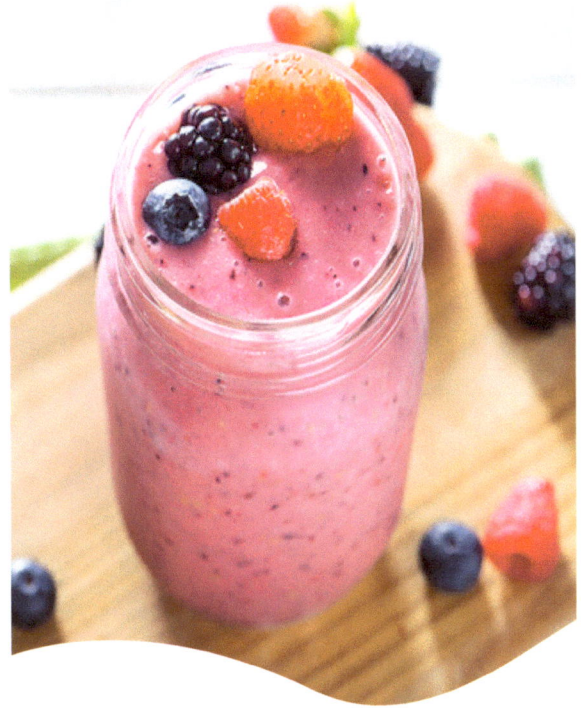

INGREDIENTS

2 cups of pitted cherries

2 cups of frozen blackberries

1 cup of frozen blueberries

1 cup of frozen raspberries

2 pitted dates (soaked) or 2 tablespoons of dried raisins (soaked)

2 cups of water

5 small kale leaves (3 kale leaves if large)

3 peppermint leaves

DIRECTIONS

Place all ingredients in a blender, process until smooth

GONE BANANAS

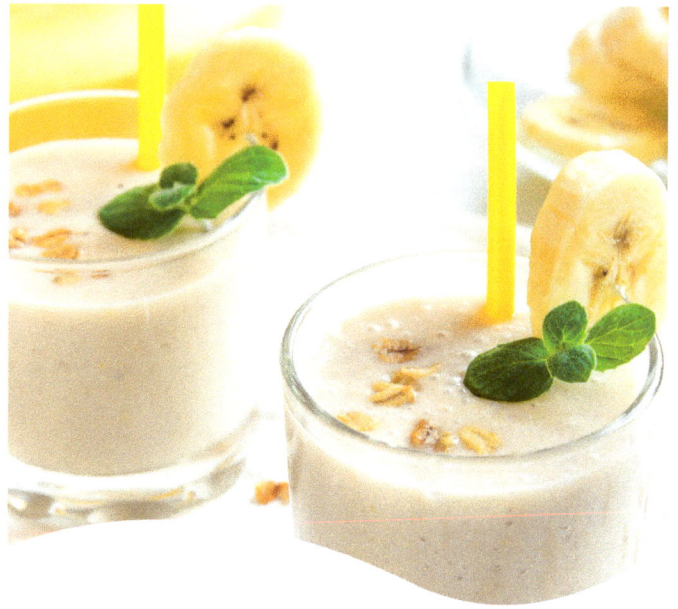

INGREDIENTS

1 yellow plantain (raw)
3 large ripe bananas
1 spoon of raisins
2 collard green leaves
2 ½ cups of water

DIRECTIONS

Soak raisins for 15 minutes in 2 ½ cups of water
Wash collard green leaves
Place all ingredients in a blender, process until smooth

FLOWING MOVEMENT

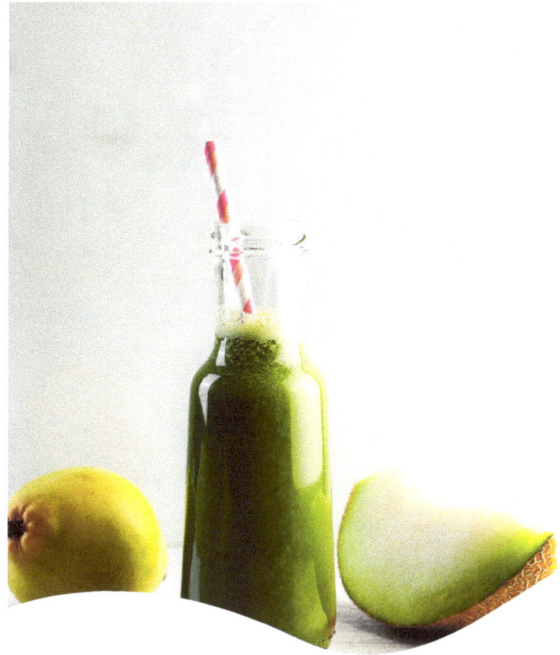

INGREDIENTS

1 pear
2 Swiss chard leaves
(remove stems)
1 cup spinach
4 pitted prunes (soaked
for 30 minutes)
1 cup water

DIRECTIONS

Place all ingredients in a blender,
process until smooth.

PINEAPPLE ORANGE ON THE GREEN

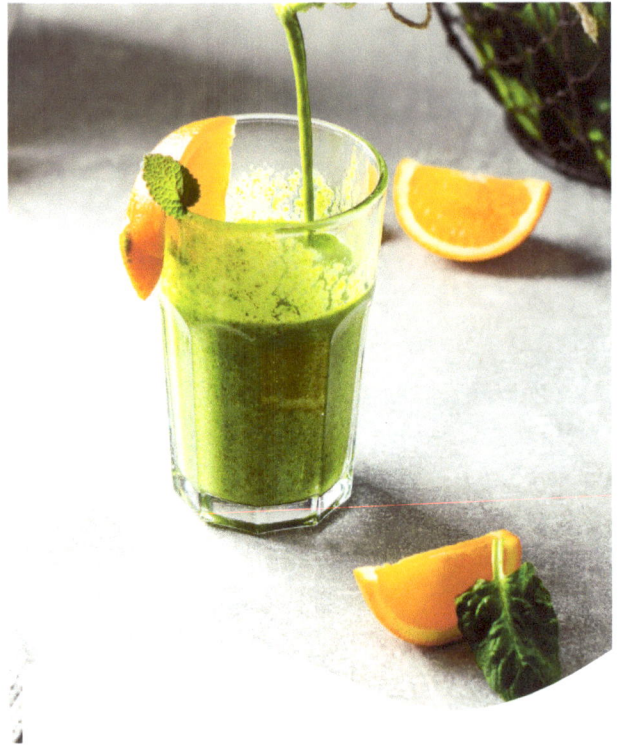

INGREDIENTS

1 orange remove seeds

1 ½ cup pineapple

½ cup water

1 cup spinach

DIRECTIONS

Place all ingredients in a blender, process until smooth.

PINA COLADA ON THE GREEN

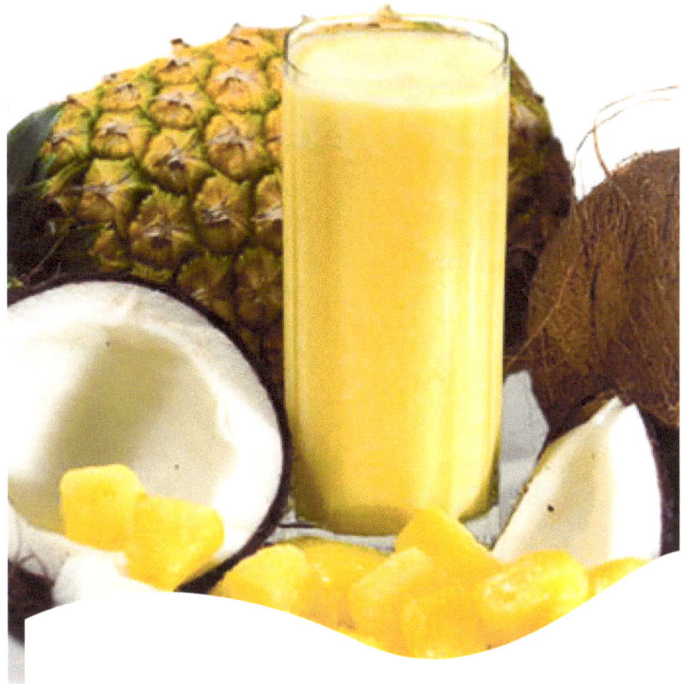

INGREDIENTS

1 ½ cup pineapple

1 cup coconut milk

1 cup spinach

DIRECTIONS

Place all ingredients in a blender, process until smooth.

VERY BERRY MOUSSE

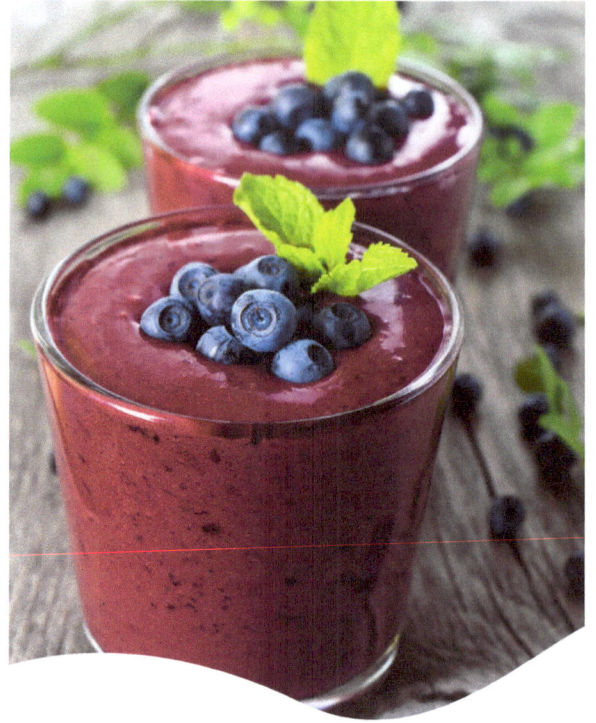

INGREDIENTS

2 ½ cups of frozen strawberries
2 ½ cups of frozen blueberries
2 ½ cups of frozen raspberries
4 to 6 pitted dates (soaked)
1 cup water

DIRECTIONS

Place all the ingredients in a blender, cover and process until smooth, pour blended mix in a glass, refrigerate for up to 1 hour, top with dates and peppermint leaf.

TROPICAL EXPLOSION

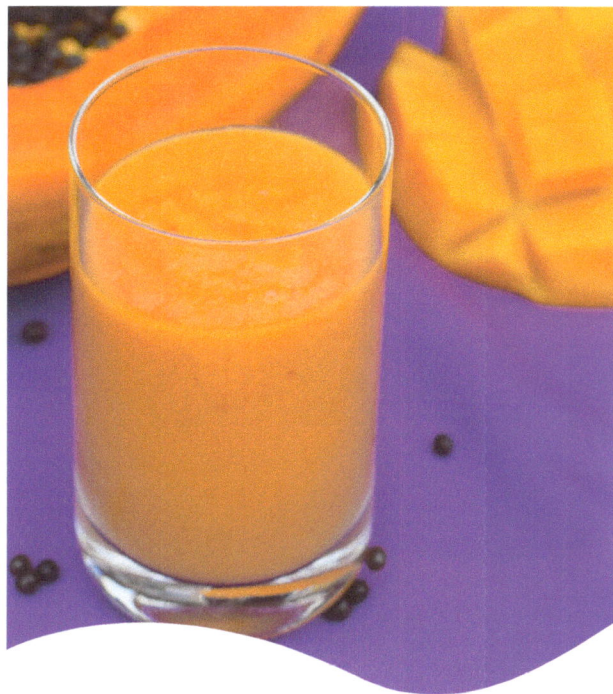

INGREDIENTS

1 ½ cup of frozen mangoes (chunks)
1 cup of fresh, chilled pineapple
2 cups of frozen papaya
1 ½ cup of water or coconut water
Nutmeg and ginger to taste

DIRECTIONS

Peel pineapple, wash collard green leaves,
place all ingredients in a blender, cover
and process until smooth

BLUEBERRY PASSION

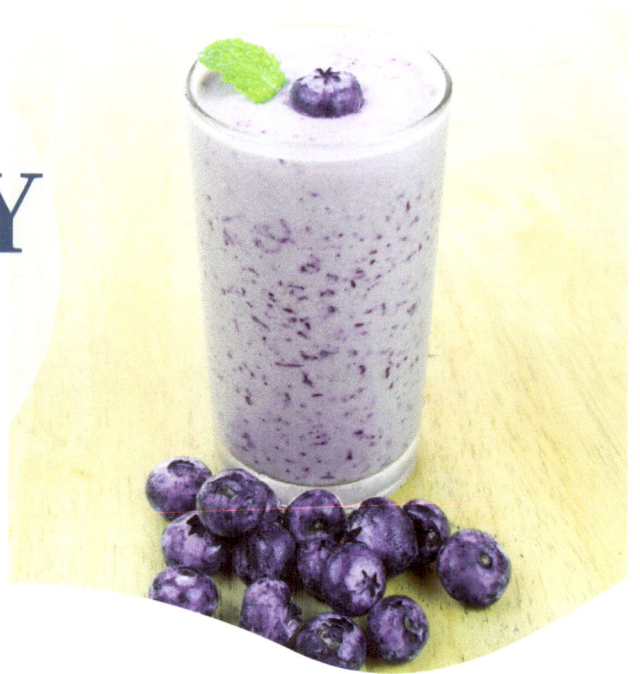

INGREDIENTS

3 kale leaves (or 4 small leaves)
1 cup frozen blueberries
1 apple
2 cups of water

DIRECTIONS

Wash apple and kale leaves, place all ingredients in a blender, cover and process until smooth

TROPICAL GREENS

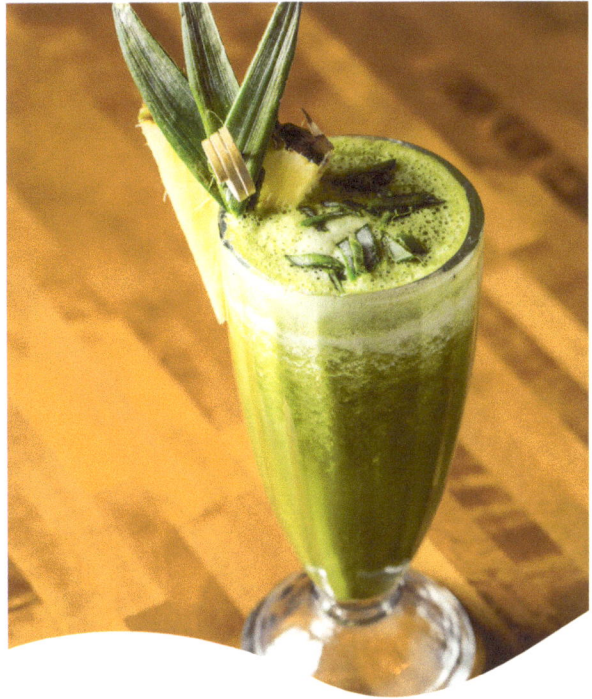

INGREDIENTS

1 cup mango (chunks)

1 cup pineapple

1 cup papaya

2 collard green leaves

2 cups of water

DIRECTIONS

Peel pineapple, wash collard green leaves, and place all ingredients in a blender, cover and process until smooth

COCONUT BREEZE

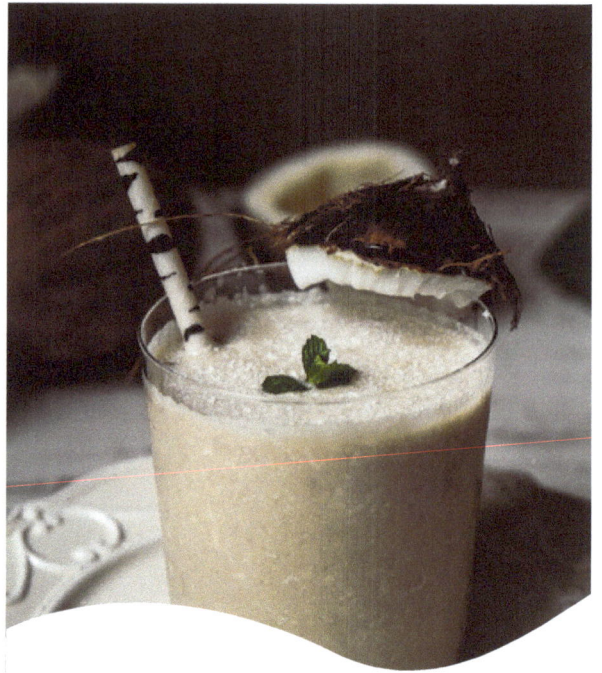

INGREDIENTS

2 young coconut meat and
water
4 ripe bananas
1/8 tea spoon nutmeg
3 drops of vanilla extract

DIRECTIONS

Place all ingredients in a blender, cover
and process until smooth

MANGO MELLOW

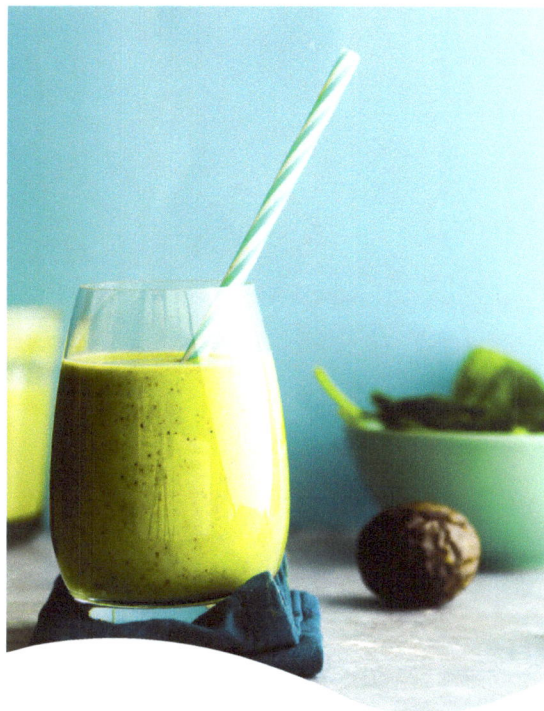

INGREDIENTS

2 cups of water
2 apples (gala)
3 cups of frozen mango
1 bunch of parsley
½ teaspoon of ground cinnamon

DIRECTIONS

Place all ingredients in a blender, cover
and process until smooth

MANGO FRESCA

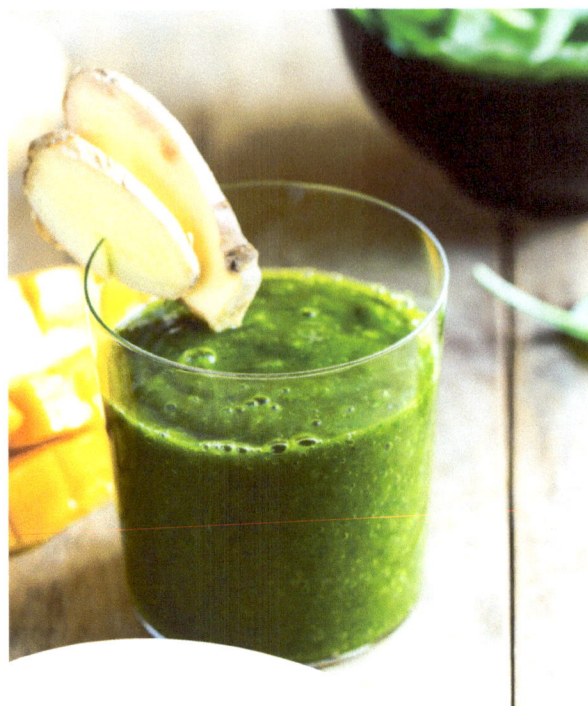

INGREDIENTS

2 cups of frozen mango
1 cup of water
1 leaf of collard green
5 peppermint leaves

DIRECTIONS

Place all ingredients in a blender, cover
and process until smooth

MANGO TONIC

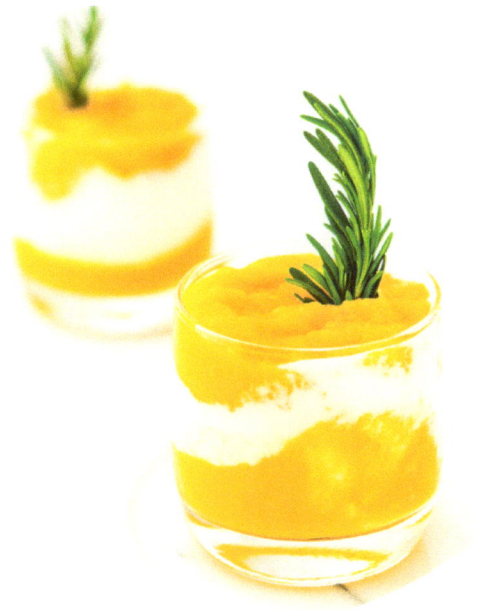

INGREDIENTS

2 cups of water from a young
coconut with meat
2 tablespoons of ground flax seeds
3 cups of frozen mango
1 cup of bok choy
1 teaspoon of moringa
1 inch of ginger
1 tablespoon of lecithin

DIRECTIONS

Place all ingredients in a blender, cover
and process until smooth

MANGO TONIC FRESCA

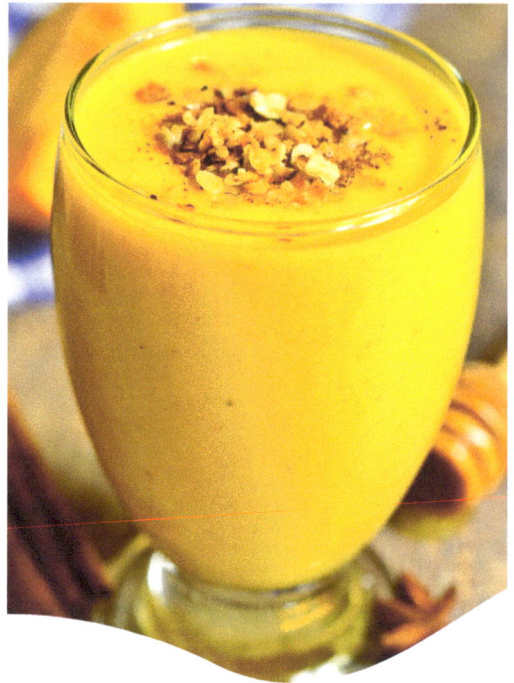

INGREDIENTS

3 cups of frozen mango
2 cups of water from a young
coconut with meat
1 cup of bok choy
1 teaspoon of moringa
2 tablespoons of ground flax seeds
1 tablespoon of lecithin
5 peppermint leaves

DIRECTIONS

Place all ingredients in a blender, cover
and process until smooth

PAPAYA TONIC

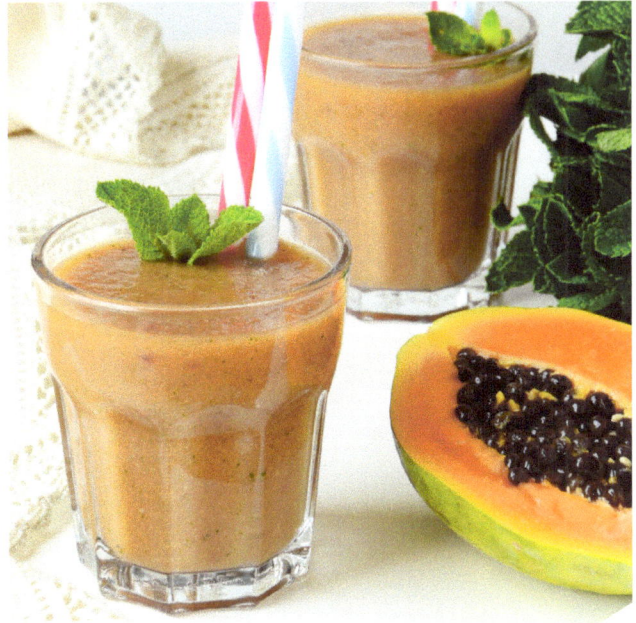

INGREDIENTS

2 cups of water from a young coconut
with meat
2 tablespoons of ground flax seeds
3 cups of frozen papaya
1 ripe banana
1 cup of swiss chard
1 teaspoon of moringa
1 inch of ginger
1 tablespoon of lecithin

DIRECTIONS

Place all ingredients in a blender, cover
and process until smooth

GONE BANANA TONIC

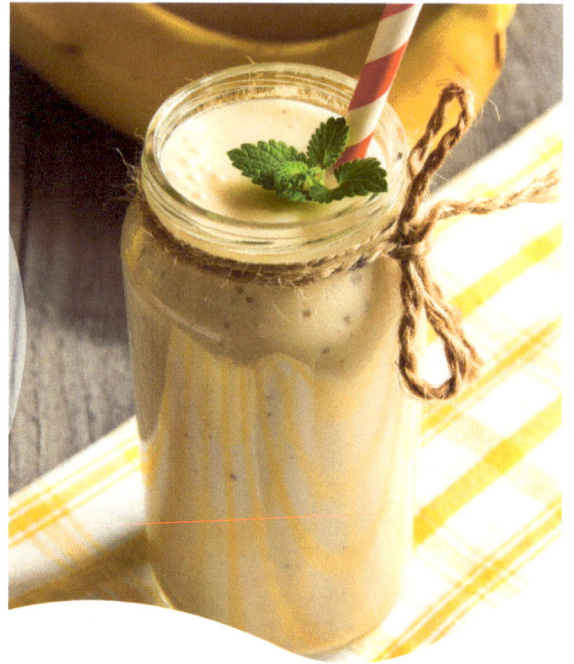

INGREDIENTS

2 cups of water from a young coconut with meat

2 tablespoons of ground flax seeds

3 ripe bananas

1 yellow plantain (raw)

1 cup of swiss chard

1 teaspoon of moringa

1 inch of ginger

1 tablespoon of soaked raisins

1 tablespoon of lecithin

DIRECTIONS

Place all ingredients in a blender, cover and process until smooth

PINEAPPLE TONIC

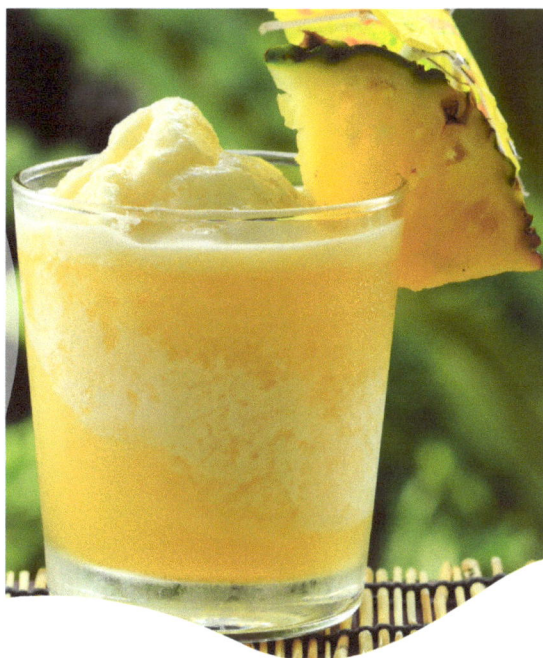

INGREDIENTS

2 cups of water from a young
coconut with meat
2 tablespoons of ground flax seeds
3 cups of frozen pineapple
1 cup of mixed green vegetables
1 teaspoon of moringa
1 inch of ginger
1 tablespoon of lecithin

DIRECTIONS

Place all ingredients in a blender, cover
and process until smooth

PINEAPPLE FRESCA

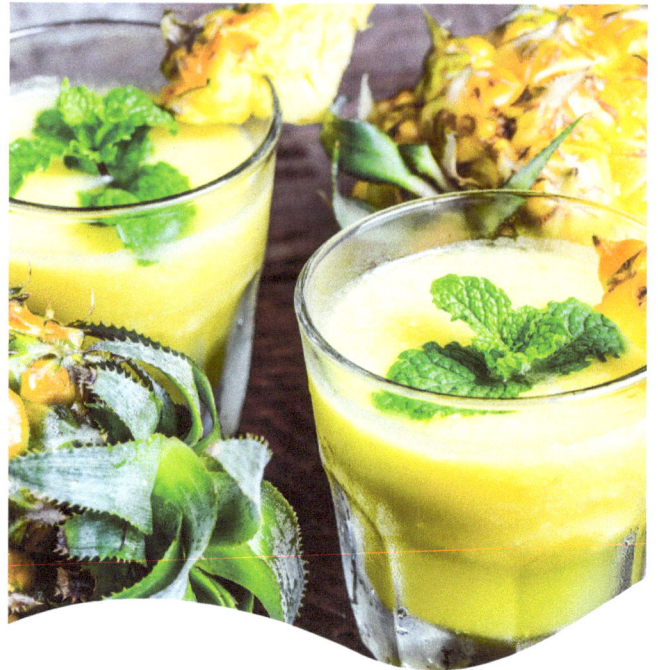

INGREDIENTS

3 cups of frozen pineapple
2 cups of water from a young
coconut with meat
1 cup of spinach
1 teaspoon of moringa
2 tablespoons of ground flax seeds
1 tablespoon of lecithin (optional)
5 peppermint leaves

DIRECTIONS

Place all ingredients in a blender, cover
and process until smooth

CARRIBEAN ALL SPICE

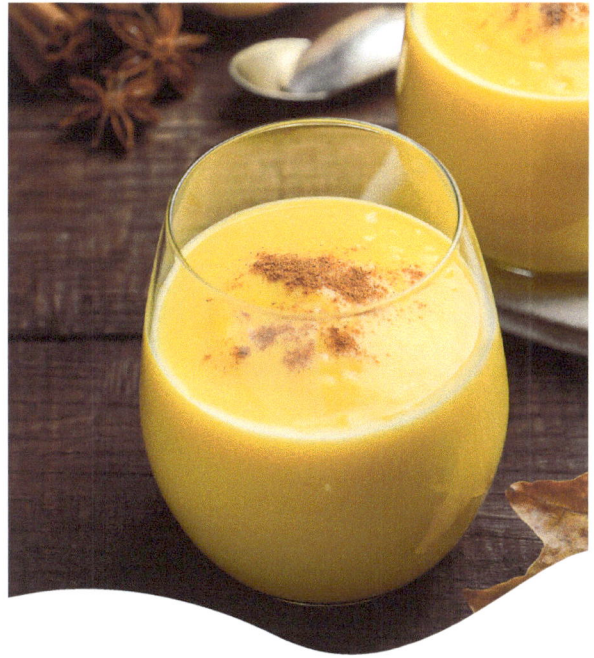

INGREDIENTS
1 cup pineapple
1 cup mango
1 cup coconut water with young
coconut meat
1 cup of butternut squash
3 tbsp. of hemp heart
Half a teaspoon of Allspice
half an inch of ginger
10 drops of vanilla extract
1 ripe banana

DIRECTIONS
Place all ingredients in a blender, cover
and process until smooth

GREEN APPLE PIE

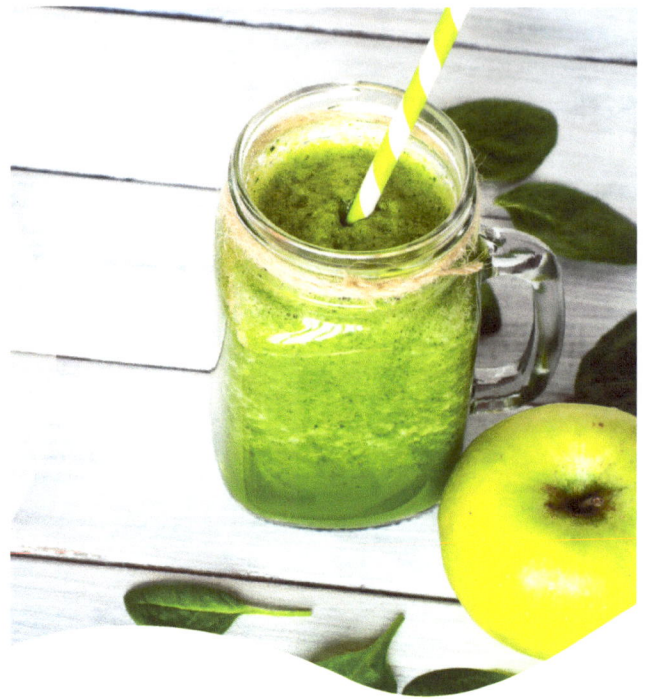

INGREDIENTS

3 apples, cored

3 frozen bananas

1 cup of spinach

4 cups nut milk (coconut)

1/4 teaspoon of cinnamon

10 drops vanilla extract

Dash of nutmeg

DIRECTIONS

Place all ingredients in a blender, cover
and process until smooth

TROPICAL SENSES

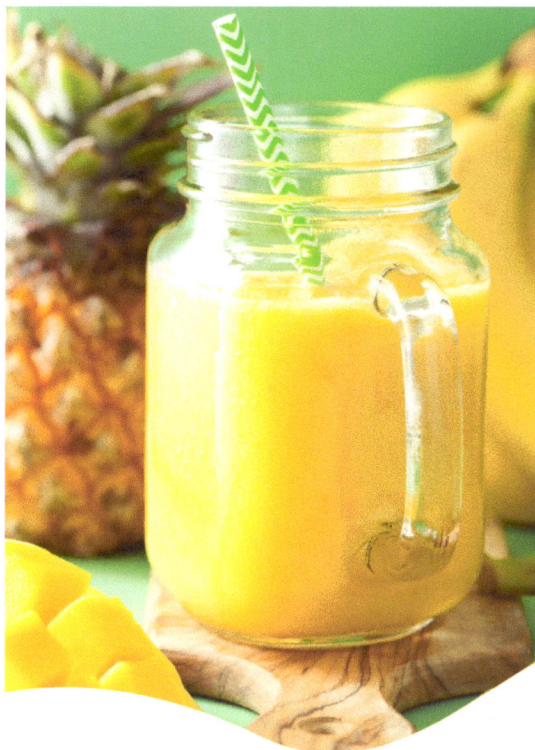

INGREDIENTS

1 cup frozen pineapple

2 cups frozen mangoes

2 cups of celery

2 cups coconut water with soft
coconut meat

1/2 inch of ginger

1/4 teaspoon allspice

10 drops of vanilla extract

DIRECTIONS

Place all ingredients in a blender, cover
and process until smooth

PURPLE BLIND DATE

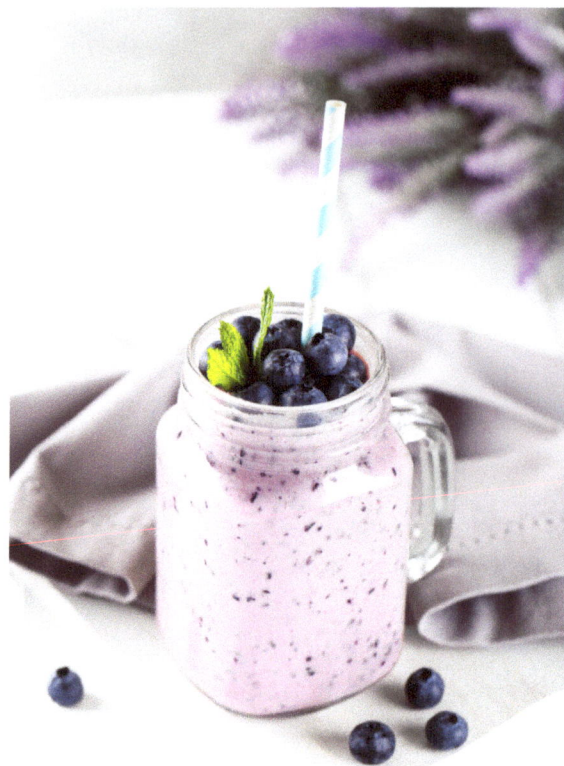

INGREDIENTS

3 kale leaves (or 6 small leaves)

2 cups frozen blueberries

2 cups coconut water

1/4 teaspoon moringa

1 teaspoon turmeric

2 tbsp hemp protein

3 dates

DIRECTIONS

Place all ingredients in a blender, cover
and process until smooth

Staying Full for Hours

Smart tips for staying full:

Don't eat so fast! Slow down and enjoy your food. Research says it takes 20 minutes for the mind to send a signal to the gut to let it know it is full. Trying to chew your food slowly can be useful also.

Consider adding ingredients like granola, chia seed, flax seeds, or hemp seeds to your smoothies. All of these ingredients are readily available in most supermarkets. Not only are they nutritious and good for you, but they add bulk to your smoothie, making it thicker and helping you stay full even longer, and help slow down how fast the body process sugar from the fruits.

ADDING SOME CRUNCH IN YOUR SMOOTHIE

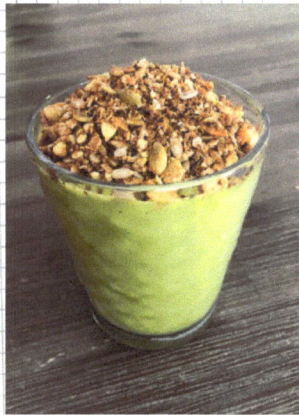

Those of you who need a little crunch in the morning, can add granola as a topping

Or, try roasted buckwheat if you prefer

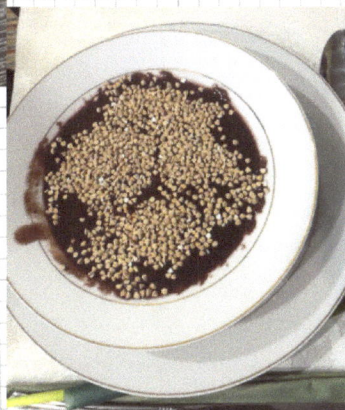

Smoothie Bowls

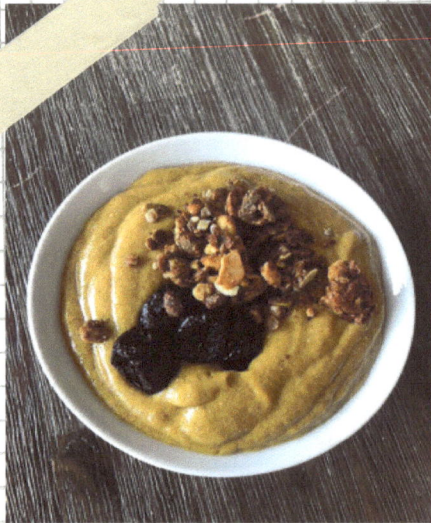

Mango, celery and water topped with prunes and grain-free granola

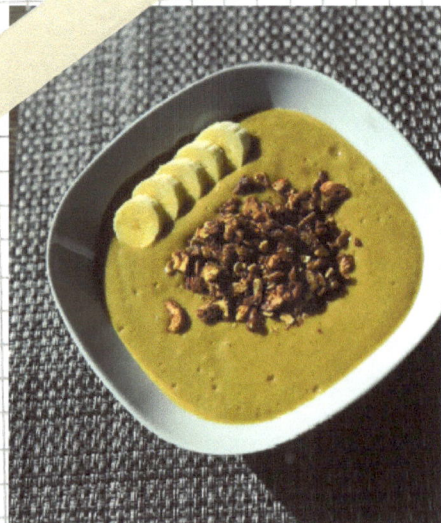

Banana, spring mix, water topped with banana and granola

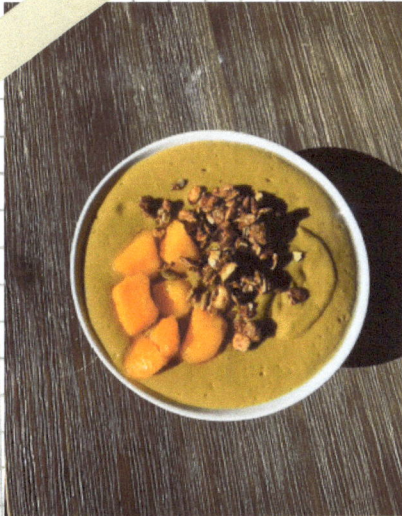

Mango, spring mix, water topped with granola and mango

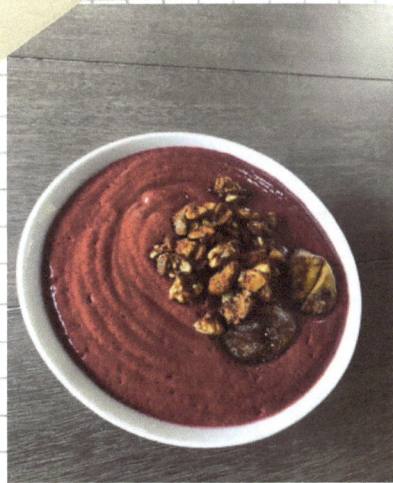

Dragon fruit, microgreens, water topped with figs and granola

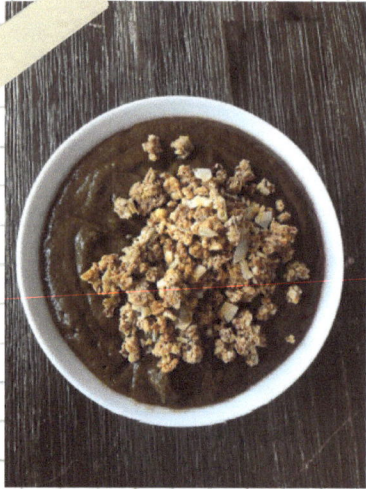

Cherries, kale topped with granola

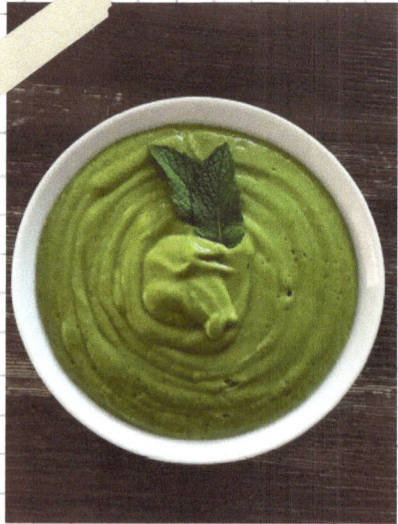

Jackfruit, spinach, peppermint and water

No Age Limit

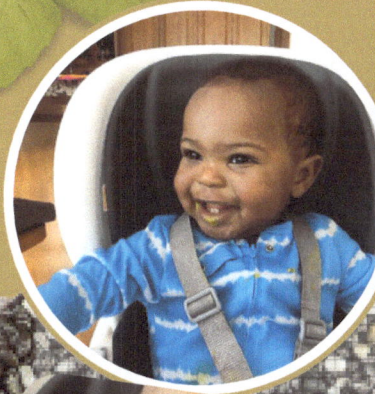

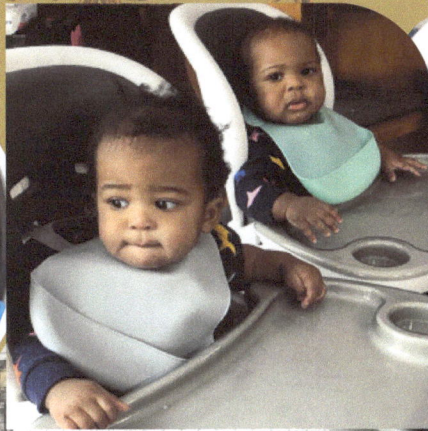

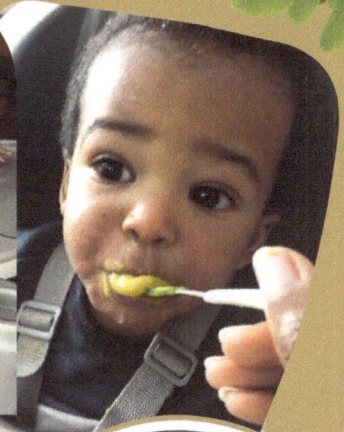

Start them young.

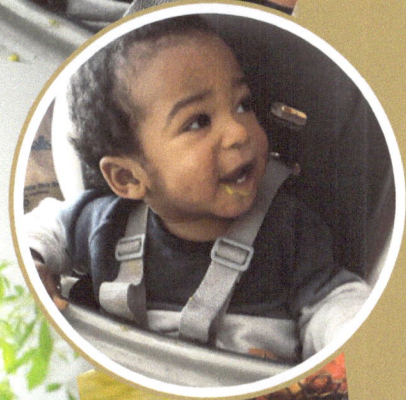

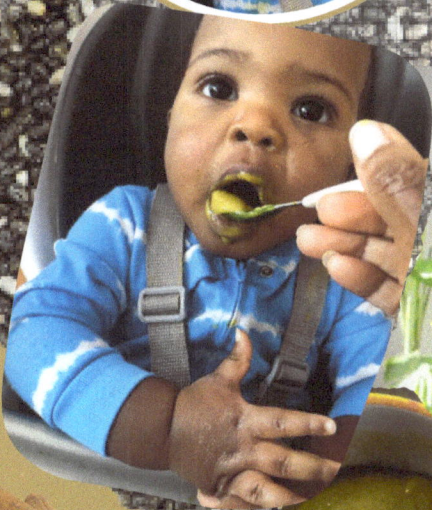

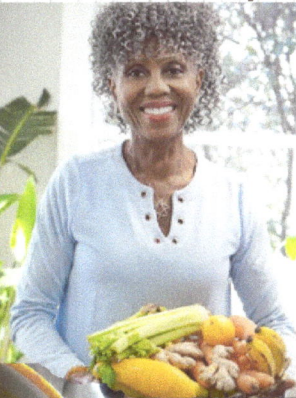

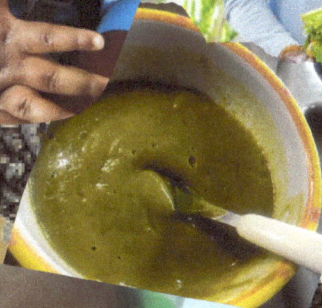

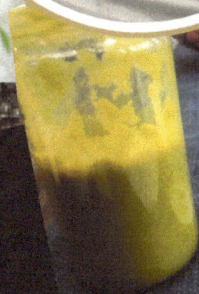

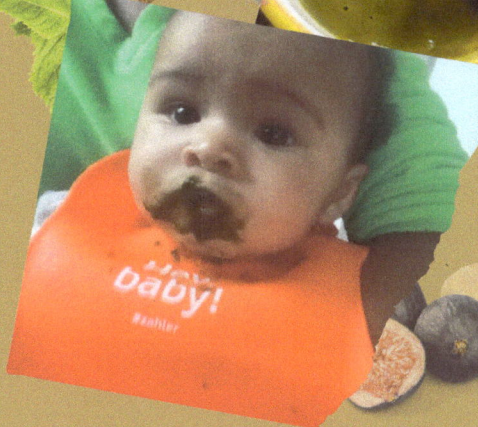

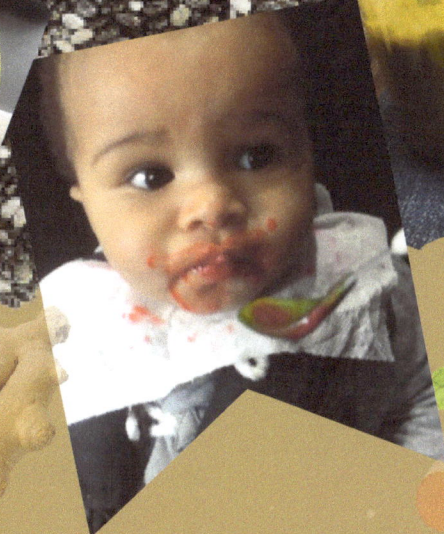

Resource Section

Get Creative with Supplements

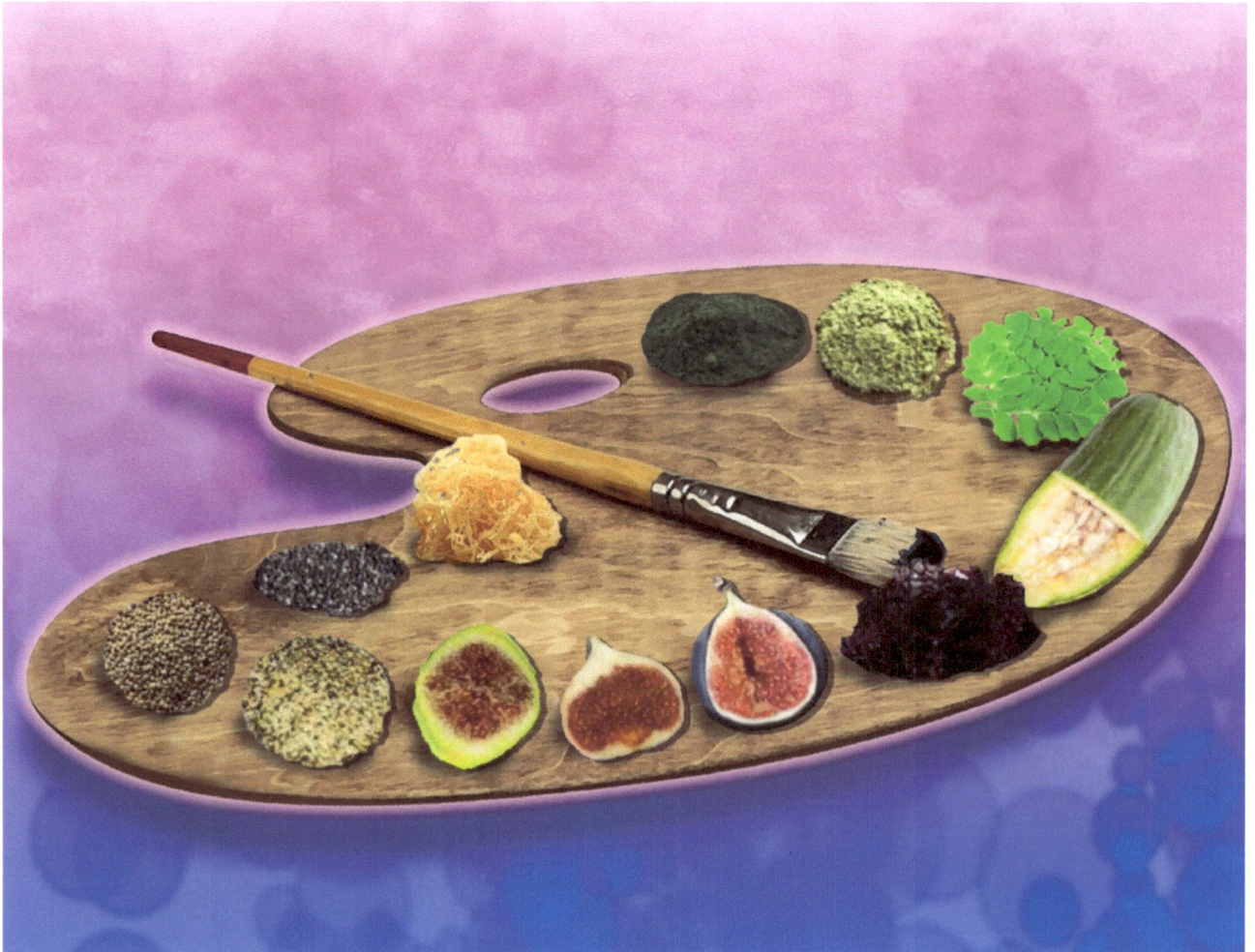

Moringa Powder

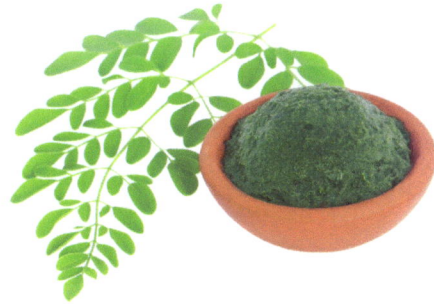

Benefits of Moringa oleifera Nourishes the Body's Immune System. Moringa oleifera provides many dozens of nutrients that strengthen your body's immune system.

Promotes Healthy Circulation. Research strongly suggests that Moringa oleifera can help support both health and function of the circulatory, blood, and cardiovascular system.

Supports Normal Blood Glucose. Moringa oleifera provides a wide array of nutrients that help normalize blood glucose levels.

Is Enzymatically Alive. Scientific research demonstrates that Moringa oleifera is rich in enzymes. Supplies Nutrients Missing in the Modern Diet. The Moringa plant provides the nutrient benefits that so many diets lack. In fact, we are receiving 75% less nutrient value for current calories consumed.

Provides Natural Anti-Aging Benefits. Moringa's wide array of antioxidant nutrients can protect the body's cells and prevent many of the common conditions associated with aging.

Delivers Anti-Inflammatory Support. Several compounds in the Moringa plant are known to support normal anti-inflammatory activity in the body.

Moringa may improve mental and cognitive clarity via many amino acids and B vitamins.

Improves your Metabolism. The nutrient benefits in Moringa provide a gentle nudge over time to improve the body's metabolic processes because of critical nutrients.

Chia seeds

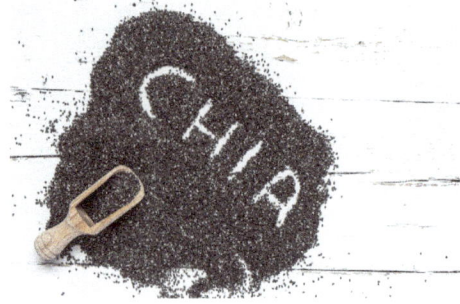

Chia seeds are very small, they are high in fiber, they are good source of calcium, iron, omega and are high in fiber.

Chia seeds is high in protein, along with a healthy balanced diet may help in controlling appetite.

Chia seeds was a staple in the Aztec and Mayan's diet to help them stay full and energized. In the Mayan language chia means strength, no wonder why I am able to go all day like an energizer bunny.

Hemp heart seeds

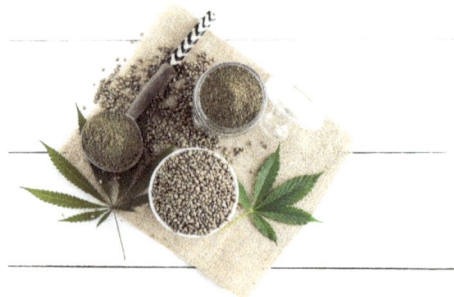

Hemp heart seeds have antioxidants and may reduce symptoms of numerous ailments, good for the heart, skin, and joints. Here are some of its nutritional benefits: Protein, which has good benefits for heart health. Fiber, may help with weight management and may stabilize blood sugar levels. Healthful fatty acids, including omega-3s and omega-6s together, may reduce inflammation. It contains vitamins and minerals such as magnesium and potassium.

Baobab

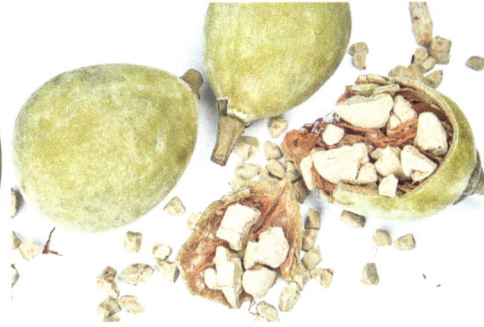

Baobab is a fruit that contains important vitamins and minerals like vitamin C, B6, magnesium, potassium, iron, prebiotic and zinc. It is high in fiber and has been shown to reduce the feeling of hunger, which may promote weight loss and may help regulate blood sugar levels. It has high fiber content, which has good benefits for digestive health. Likewise, it may decrease levels of inflammation in the body due to its antioxidant and polyphenols properties. Furthermore, Baobab whether consumed fresh or in powder is packed with nutritional benefits when consumed or added to food and drinks.

Irish Sea Moss

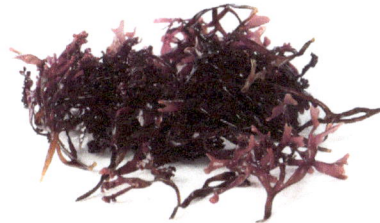

Scientific Name: Chondrus crispus, known under these names also: Sea Moss, Carrageen Moss, Irish Moss. This food from the sea varies in color from white to purple or orange, the variation in color does not affect their phytochemical value.
Sea Moss is naturally raw, wild crafted and sundried.

Irish Sea Moss has been consumed for a long time throughout the world; research indicates that this sea vegetable is loaded with minerals; it is also a good source of B vitamins, vitamin C and Beta Carotene.

Blue-Green Algae

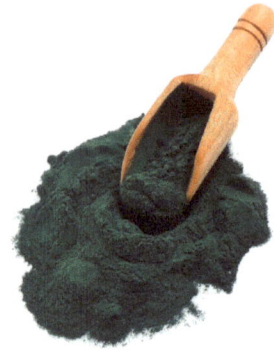

Blue-green algae belong to a group of bacteria that naturally grows in marine and freshwater systems. It's a good source of protein, iron, and small amounts of vitamins C, E, and folate. It contains beta-carotene and other minerals. Furthermore, it is used to assist in treating high blood pressure, diabetes, and obesity. Blue-green algae is also used as a supplement which may help in losing weight. In addition it may help to boost the immune system and control cholesterol levels.

Figs

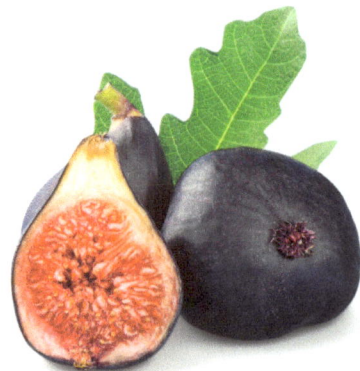

Scientific name: Ficus carica known as figs. Inside are tiny seeds, and an edible purple or green peel. It has a mild sweet taste and pink flesh. Figs are nutritious fruit high in calcium, potassium, copper, vitamin B6 and fiber. Fresh figs contain some calories from natural sugar, while dried figs contain high sugar and are rich in calories. The fruit and leaves are packed with a variety of health benefits for the body.

Herbal Addition

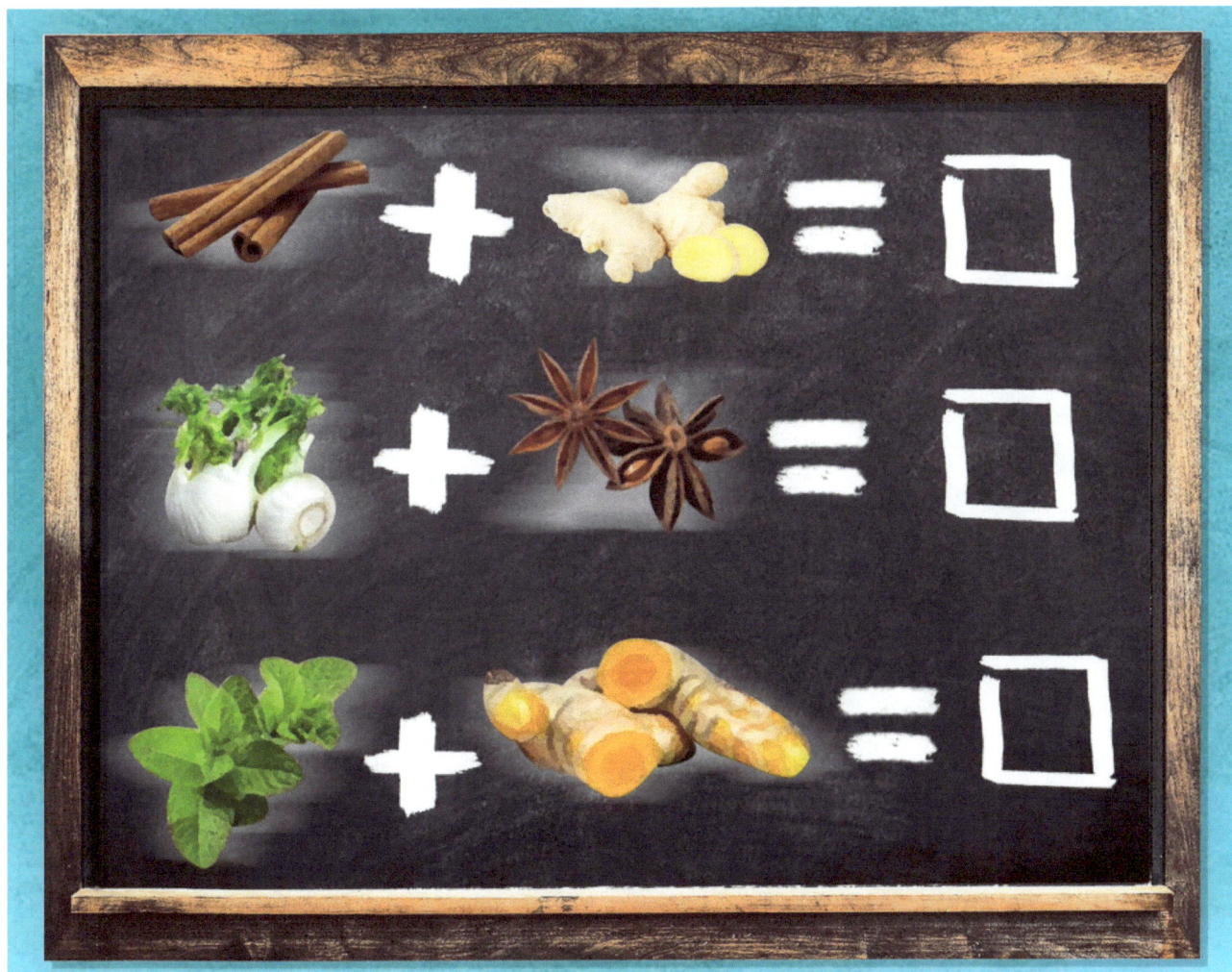

Turmeric

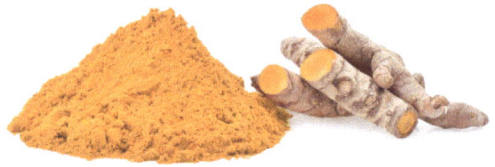

Turmeric comes from the rootstock of the Curcuma longa plant, which comes from the ginger family.

Turmeric has been used to treat different diseases, including cancer and skin infections.

It has anti-inflammatory and antiseptic properties used to treat wounds and infections. Turmeric gradually increases antioxidants in the body, helps lower cholesterol, and may help people with depression.

Caution: Refrain from using turmeric prior to any surgical intervention including tooth extraction; turmeric may cause excessive bleeding.

Cinnamon

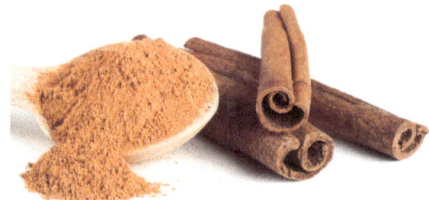

Cinnamon has anti-inflammatory properties that may help fight body infection, antimicrobial, antioxidant, antitumor, cardiovascular, cholesterol-lowering, and immunomodulatory effects.

Adding cinnamon to your diet may lower blood sugar due to its powerful anti-diabetic effect. It can be added to foods, and drinks and is used in cooking and baking. One of the most active ingredients in cinnamon is cinnamaldehyde that is used in flavorings and fragrances.

Peppermint

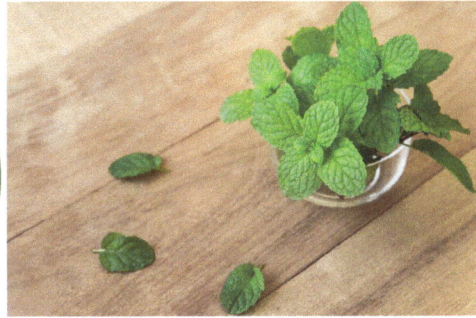

Peppermint or Mentha x piperita is an aromatic plant used to add flavor or fragrance to foods, drinks, toothpaste, mouthwashes, soaps, cosmetics, and some medicinal uses. The leaf and oil are used as medicine. Peppermint may help people with indigestion, bedsores, headache, anxiety, and insomnia. Menthol, the main chemical component of peppermint, is an effective decongestant used for colds and cough.

Spearmint

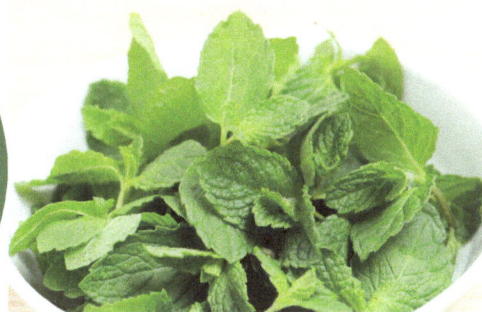

Scientific name: Mentha Spicata or spearmint comes from the mint plant. Its name is from its characteristic spear-shaped leaves. Spearmint leaves and essential oils are used as a flavoring in foods, drinks and cosmetics. It has a sweet taste and is used to flavor toothpaste, mouthwash, candy, and chewing gum. Its leaves can be made into tea.

Basil

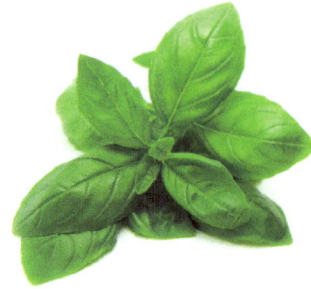

Scientific name: Ocimum basilicum is a culinary herb of the family Lamiaceae. Basil is a leafy green herb that originated in Asia and Africa. It's a member of the mint family and is often used in cuisines due to its aromatic and flavorful characteristics. Its leaves are also used in teas and supplements that may have good health benefits.

Basil has many varieties. Sweet basil is the most popular that is sold dried in supermarkets. Bush or greek basil, has a strong aroma yet mild flavor and can be a substitute for sweet basil.

Thai basil has an anise-licorice flavor commonly used in Thai and Southeast Asian dishes. Cinnamon basil has a cinnamon-like flavor and scent. Lettuce basil has large, wrinkled, soft leaves with a licorice-like flavor and is great for salads

Fennel

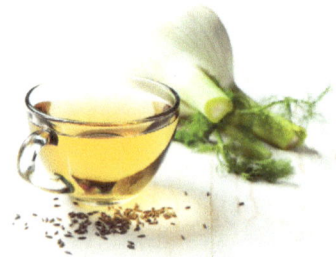

Fennel or Foeculum Vulgare is a flowering plant species in the carrot family. Its dried seeds are used in food and oils are used as medicine. It is a flavorful herb used in some cuisines. Its bulb and seeds have a mild, licorice-like flavor. Fennel and its seeds are known to have health benefits and may provide anti-oxidant, anti-inflammatory, and anti-bacterial effects. It may also suppress appetite and may relieve mild constipation

Star Anise

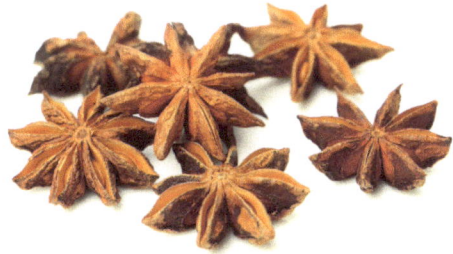

Anise, also called Pimpinella Anisum, is an herb that is from the same family as carrots and celery. It is used to add flavors to foods, beverages, candies, breath fresheners, and fragrances in soap. The root and leaf are used for medicine. It has anti-fungal, anti-viral; and anti-bacterial properties. Star anise is a popular ingredient in some cuisines and can be added to soup and drinks.

Ginger

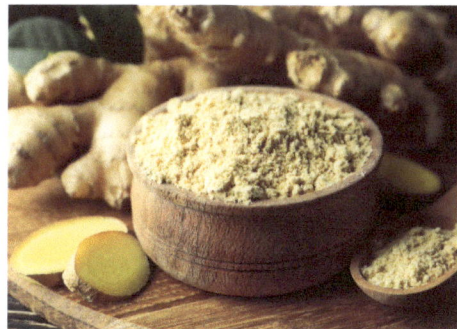

Ginger is a flowering plant whose root is used as a spice and medicine. It is widely used in cooking and sometimes added to processed foods. Its fragrance and flavor come from its natural oil, which has anti-inflammatory, anti-diabetic, and antioxidant effects. It may treat nausea and may help in losing weight. It has been shown that using ginger may lower blood sugar levels and help people with indigestion.

Caution: Refrain from using ginger prior to any surgical intervention including tooth extraction; ginger may cause excessive bleeding.

Resources

Moringa Super-Food
Where to find it:
https://yesicanseminars.com/

Chia Seeds
Where to find it: Amazon, local supermarket

Hemp heart seeds
Where to find it: Amazon

Baobab
Where to find it:
https://yesicanseminars.com/product/baobab-andansonia-digitata-12oz/

Irish Sea Moss
Where to find it:
https://yesicanseminars.com/product/irish-seamoss/

Blue-Green Algae
Where to find it: Amazon, health food store

Figs
Where to find it: Amazon, local supermarket

Turmeric
Where to find it: Amazon, local supermarket

Cinnamon
Where to find it: Amazon, local supermarket

Peppermint
Where to find it: Amazon, local supermarket, home garden

Spearmint
Where to find it: Amazon, local supermarket, home garden

Basil
Where to find it: Amazon, local supermarket

Fennel
Where to find it: Amazon, local supermarket

Star Anise
Where to find it: Amazon, local supermarket

Ginger
Where to find it: Amazon, local supermarket

To learn more about conventional and organic produce, labels, and pesticide residues visit Consumer Reports and the Environmental Work Group at:
https://www.consumerreports.org &
https://www.ewg.org/foodnews/

Blender Resources

Blender Resources

High Speed Blender: Vitamix
High Speed Blender: Blendtec
Blender: Osterizer
Blender: Hamilton Beach
Mini Blender: Nutri Bullet
Travel Blender: Nutri Bullet
Travel Size Portable Blender: Nutri Bullet Go,
Hamilton Beach, One Speed, Blendjet

Making smoothies has never been easier!

Don't have much time at home? With a portable blender, you can't make excuses for not being able to make your smoothie every day. Whether you're at work, at a dorm, or traveling on vacation, you can bring one anywhere.

You can have all the tools to take it to the finish line. So get yourself a portable blender if needed.

Words of Wisdom:

"Don't go out and buy an expensive blender if you are not sure you are committed to this lifestyle."

YOU DID IT!

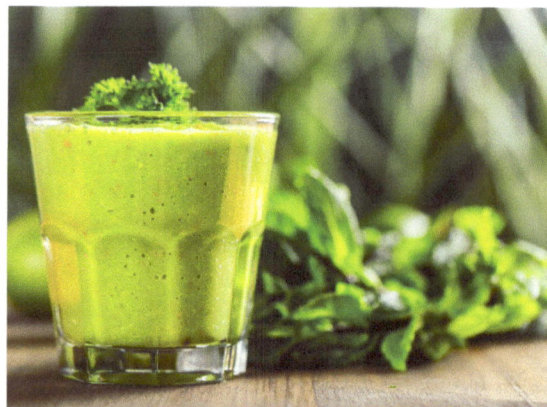

Congratulations on finishing your 40 days detox smoothies challenge. Continue to keep up this routine and feel good for life!

As I mentioned in the beginning, drinking green smoothies each morning has contributed to my vitality at 66 years old and counting. Since then, I feel more energetic and strong all day, I rarely get sick, I have a sharp mind, and I am able to keep up with my four-year-old granddaughter Maya and my eighteen month-old twin grandsons, Myles and Tyson. I always stay productive. I'm confident that drinking green smoothies will do the same to you!

Did you feel like you were making progress with positive adjustments but needed more assistance or guidance? Feel free to email me with any questions at info@yesicanseminars.com

Feel free to inquire about our 3 months, 6 months or 12 months program
www.yesicanseminars.com

We would love to see your smoothie creations! Share pictures of your taste treats on social channels.
Be sure to tag us and use the #40DaySmoothiebyYICS
Join our Facebook group

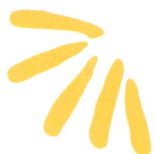

@yesicanseminars or yesicandoit2
Yes I Can Seminars, LLC

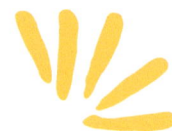

"Take care of your body. It's the only place you have to live."

-JIM ROHN

Finish Line

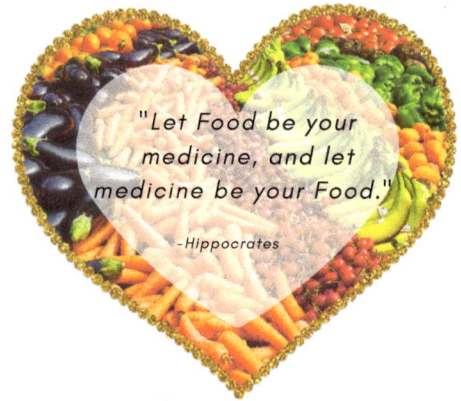

"Let Food be your medicine, and let medicine be your Food."

-Hippocrates

Now that you have made it to the finish line, what are your plans moving forward?

Please go back to your daily journal and take one last look at the benefits, what you enjoyed, and the smoothies that you felt won your heart. Then, take a few minutes to create a short plan to move forward with a wellness recipe that you can easily follow.

Planning is the key to success. Most people miss the finish line because they failed to plan.

Book a Free 15 minutes strategy session for massive results
www.yesicanseminars.com

yes I Can

LET ME SHOW YOU HOW TO TRANSFORM YOURSELF

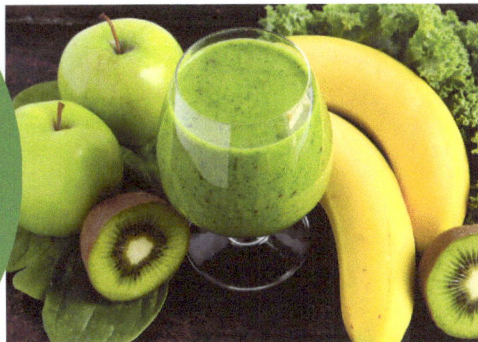

1995 180 pounds

2004 140 pounds

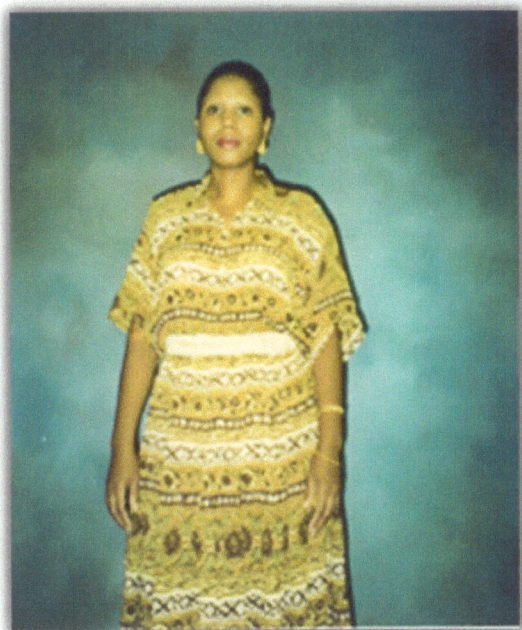

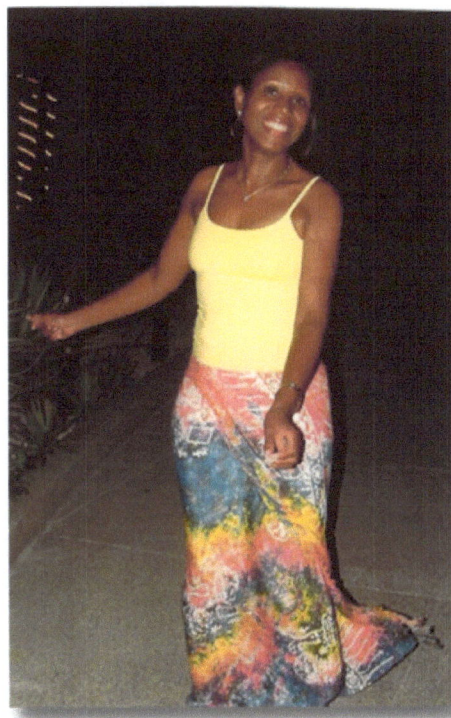

TESTIMONIALS

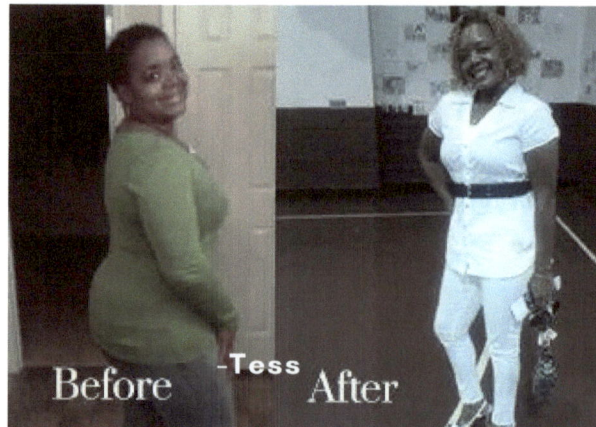

Before -Tess After

Yep – I did it – FINALLY. Can't say it was easy. It was a lot of hard work and determination. I just wanted to say thanks again for all your help.

Tess

This whole experience has been an eye opener, lifestyle changing experience for me. If it has not been for this Mindset Lifestyle Change it would not be possible. I feel that through this Lifestyle Change will save my life!!!

Yvonne

This Lifestyle has made me healthier than I have ever been in my life. I feel and look wonderful and so happy that I got the opportunity to have Immacula in my life. She has inspired me to keep fit and keep myself in shape.

Jennifer

I admit that I never really did your plan. Well, I found it again on Sunday after having mentally changed my food mindset. I am doing really well with it. I am full and satisfied. I already feel the benefits of this life change and plan to stick to it. Thank you so much for the direction. I should have done this long ago.

Diane

When I began this journey I saw significant improvements in my skin not to mention the increase in energy and mental vitality.
I have come to incorporate healthier foods into my diet, including more fruits, vegetables and grains.
I view this change as a lifestyle and not just a short term goal, Immacula was very instrumental in recommending substitutes for the things I love, which has helped me to stay on course. Also as a bonus allergies and stuffy nose are a thing of the past. I would definitely recommend her services to anyone.

Akia

Immacula Oligario has been a great inspiration and a role model for me. Her emotional and spiritual support through the hard times has always helped me stay focused on my goals. The example that I have set for my children gives me a sense of achievement that has filled my life with joy.

MaryAnn

Immacula was careful to listen to every detail and document all that I had to tell her. I began the journey thinking "who am I kidding, I can't do this." Now when I look back this has been a total transformation.

Immacula has been there for the good, bad, highs, lows, late night conversations of encouragement and answering questions. I now have a renewed sense of self. I have so much energy, drive and determination.

Philesha

I must have a cup of coffee every morning in order to function at optimal capacity. That's what I thought until I tried Immacula's detox program. The additional fiber in my diet keeps things moving through the colon. it gives you the nutrients that the body needs while eliminating what the body does not need. It works! I have never felt better.

Dr. Sherry

My Journey towards Freedom...

I am a 34 year old pre-diabetic wife and mother of a one year old, my daughter is the main reason why made a decision to address my addiction; I want to set better example for her and be healthy.

I now am a woman who has a new determination to live life with understanding and new tools to help propel me to FREEDOM from food addiction.

Amanda

The day I let go of denial was the day I called Immacula. My life was unbalanced and the scales had begun to show signs of tilting. Through coaching and consultations with Immacula, I've learned positive re-enforcement, healthy body concepts and stress relieving techniques.

Crystal

Immacula's approach to the life style change was not a hard sell. It was her genuine concern for my health as well as her willingness to share information. Thank you Immacula for your concern advice and continued support.

Glenn

I attended one of Immacula's retreats for healthier eating and at first I was skeptical. I thought I would feel hungry and weak but I woke up singing, "I feel good!"

Diana

I was faced with a health challenge. Immacula invited me to a weekend retreat the results are tremendous... more energy... weight control... clearer skin... regulated bowels. I went from an unbelieving physician to a converted physician. Thank you Immacula for caring about my life!

Dr. Nixon

With an open mind & dedication, we can retrain our taste buds to break eating habits of certain types of food that we are used to which are toxic. We can be sure to achieve successful changes.

Sharllee

SHOPPING LIST

VEGETABLES

- [ ] Spinach
- [ ] Celery
- [ ] Lettuce
- [ ] Collard greens
- [ ] Swiss chard
- [ ] Butternut
- [ ] squash
- [ ] Bok choy
- [ ] Kale

FROZEN

- [ ] Strawberry
- [ ] Raspberry
- [ ] Blueberry
- [ ] Bananas
- [ ] Pineapple
- [ ] Blackberry
- [ ] Papaya

MISCELANIOUS

- [ ] Raisins
- [ ] Dates
- [ ] Prunes
- [ ] Coconut meat

FRUITS

- [ ] Mango
- [ ] Orange
- [ ] Coconut
- [ ] Pineapple
- [ ] Strawberry
- [ ] Banana
- [ ] Cherry
- [ ] Blackberry
- [ ] Blueberry
- [ ] Raspberry
- [ ] Yellow plantain
- [ ] Pear
- [ ] Dates
- [ ] Papaya
- [ ] Apple
- [ ] Dragon fruit
- [ ] Jackfruit

LIQUIDS

- [ ] Coconut milk
- [ ] Coconut water
- [ ] Vanilla extract
- [ ] Almond milk
- [ ] Rice milk
- [ ] Hemp milk
- [ ] Oat milk
- [ ] Plain water

HERBS & SPICES

- [ ] Cinnamon
- [ ] Peppermint
- [ ] Nutmeg
- [ ] Ginger
- [ ] Vanilla
- [ ] Parsley
- [ ] Flax seeds
- [ ] Lecithin
- [ ] Ginger
- [ ] Mint
- [ ] Fennel
- [ ] Allspice
- [ ] Star anise
- [ ] Basil
- [ ] Spearmint
- [ ] Turmeric
- [ ] Figs
- [ ] Bluegreen algae
- [ ] Irish sea moss
- [ ] Baobab
- [ ] Hemp heart seeds
- [ ] Chia seeds
- [ ] Moringa powder

CEREAL

- [ ] Granola
- [ ] Buckwheat

It is a greater disappointment to get home from the grocery store to find out that you are missing ingredients to get prepared for your week. I highly recommend that you use the shopping list provided above to ensure that you are ready to transform or supercharge you life.

This book is a wonderful companion to our Smoothie Detox Reset Challenge Program which is our Next Level 5 week group challenge.
Each week will be a step in the direction of your goal.

WEEK 1

40-Day Detox Reset +Action flow

- Where are you and where do you want to be?
- Where are you on your journey?
- What is your expectation for this journey?
- Do you have a plan to get there?
- Diet VS Lifestyle
- Getting to Know you
- Take Control of your wheel
- Your family tree

WEEK 2

Your Road Map + Action Plan

- Introduction to green smoothies and their benefits
- How to create delicious green smoothies
- Benefits of drinking green smoothies
- Mixology
- What are green smoothies?
- Do you know your fruit and vegetables?
- Create your road map

WEEK 3

- Understanding GMO
- Negative effects of toxins
- How toxins affect us
- How to keep them out
- How toxins contribute to weight gain
- Importance of keeping liver clean in weight loss
- How to cleanse liver

WEEK 4

- Smoothie making tips
- Smoothie preparation and storing
- Blender choice
- BPA safety
- Inclusion not seclusion
- Setting yourself for a successful journey
- Daily planner
- Daily Journal
- Track your favorite

WEEK 5

- How to supercharge your smoothie
- Superfoods
- Herbs
- Healthy lifestyle tips
- How to create sustainable energy and vitality
- You did it!
- You are at the finish line
- Bonus

Visit www.yesicanseminars.com to learn more

Next level is Detox Made Easy

©Detox
Reset
CHALLENGE

Your Road to Better Health and Permanent Weight Loss

Simple steps to losing weight and keeping it off for good!!!

Are you looking to:
- Lose weight and keep it off?
- Have energy all day?
- Eat foods you enjoy?
- Stop depriving yourself with diet?
- Feel better about the person you see in the mirror?
- Look and feel sexy?
- Have self-confidence and self-esteem?

Are you that kind of person who wants to feel great everyday?

You are in the right place!
Being healthy doesn't have to be challenging.
This detox reset challenge program offers you boundless energy, clearer skin, better sleep, less stress, less health concerns...

JOIN OUR FACEBOOK GROUP NOW AND FOLLOW US ON INSTAGRAM!!!!!

40-DAY DETOX RESET CHALLENGE-Yes I Can Seminars
@yesicanseminars

SEASONAL DETOX

I invite you to start your road to better health!

Starting your road to better health has countless benefits, which includes permanent weight loss.

Consider trying our seasonal detox program, which offers tailored detox options for spring, summer, fall, and winter.

Each season presents unique challenges to our bodies, and our program is designed to support your body's natural detoxification processes through a combination of nourishing foods and healthy habits.

More information to come in our second book, "Detox Made Easy".

www.ingramcontent.com/pod-product-compliance
Lightning Source LLC
Chambersburg PA
CBHW060858270326
41935CB00003B/24